Controversies in Spinal and Cranial Surgery

Editors

RUSSELL R. LONSER
DANIEL K. RESNICK

NEUROSURGERY CLINICS OF NORTH AMERICA

www.neurosurgery.theclinics.com

Consulting Editors
RUSSELL R. LONSER
DANIEL K. RESNICK

July 2017 • Volume 28 • Number 3

ELSEVIER

1600 John F. Kennedy Boulevard • Suite 1800 • Philadelphia, Pennsylvania, 19103-2899

http://www.theclinics.com

NEUROSURGERY CLINICS OF NORTH AMERICA Volume 28, Number 3
July 2017 ISSN 1042-3680, ISBN-13: 978-0-323-53140-5

Editor: Stacy Eastman
Developmental Editor: Colleen Dietzler

Neurosurgery Clinics of North America (ISSN 1042-3680) is published quarterly by Elsevier Inc., 360 Park Avenue South, New York, NY 10010-1710. Months of issue are January, April, July, and October. Business and Editorial Offices: 1600 John F. Kennedy Blvd., Suite 1800, Philadelphia, PA 19103-2899. Customer Service Office: 11830 Westline Industrial Drive, St. Louis, MO 63146. Periodicals postage paid at New York, NY, and additional mailing offices. Subscription prices are $393.00 per year (US individuals), $665.00 per year (US institutions), $423.00 per year (Canadian individuals), $826.00 per year (Canadian institutions), $505.00 per year (international individuals), $826.00 per year (international institutions), $100.00 per year (US students), and $255.00 per year (international and Canadian students). International air speed delivery is included in all *Clinics* subscription prices. All prices are subject to change without notice. **POSTMASTER:** Send address changes to *Neurosurgery Clinics of North America*, Elsevier Periodicals Customer Service, 11830 Westline Industrial Drive, St. Louis, MO 63146. **Customer Service: 1-800-654-2452 (US and Canada). From outside the US and Canada, call: 1-314-453-7041. Fax: 1-314-453-5170. E-mail: JournalsCustomerService-usa@elsevier.com (for print support) and journalsonlinesupport-usa@elsevier.com (for online support).**

Reprints. For copies of 100 or more, of articles in this publication, please contact the Commercial Reprints Department, Elsevier Inc., 360 Park Avenue South, New York, NY 10010-1710. Tel. 212-633-3874; Fax: 212-633-3820; E-mail: reprints@elsevier.com.

Neurosurgery Clinics of North America is covered in *MEDLINE/PubMed (Index Medicus), EMBASE/Excerpta Medica, and Current Contents/Clinical Medicine (CC/CM).*

Contributors

CONSULTING EDITORS

RUSSELL R. LONSER, MD
Professor and Chair, Dardinger Family Chair
in Oncological Neurosurgery, Department of
Neurological Surgery, The Ohio State
University Wexner Medical Center, Columbus,
Ohio

DANIEL K. RESNICK, MD, MS
Professor and Vice Chairman for Academic
Affairs, Residency Program Director,
Department of Neurological Surgery,
Professor, Department of Orthopedics and
Rehabilitation Medicine, Co-Director, Spine
Surgery Program, University of Wisconsin
School of Medicine and Public Health,
Madison, Wisconsin

EDITORS

RUSSELL R. LONSER, MD
Professor and Chair, Dardinger Family Chair
in Oncological Neurosurgery, Department of
Neurological Surgery, The Ohio State
University Wexner Medical Center, Columbus,
Ohio

DANIEL K. RESNICK, MD, MS
Professor and Vice Chairman for Academic
Affairs, Residency Program Director,
Department of Neurological Surgery,
Professor, Department of Orthopedics and
Rehabilitation Medicine, Co-Director, Spine
Surgery Program, University of Wisconsin
School of Medicine and Public Health,
Madison, Wisconsin

AUTHORS

RAMI JAMES N. AOUN, MD, MPH
Department of Neurological Surgery, Precision
Neuro-therapeutics Innovation Lab,
Neurosurgery Simulation and Innovation Lab,
Mayo Clinic Hospital, Mayo Clinic, Phoenix,
Arizona

JEFFREY S. BEECHER, DO
Endovascular Neurosurgery Fellow,
Department of Neurosurgery, Jacobs School
of Medicine and Biomedical Sciences,
University at Buffalo, State University of
New York, Gates Vascular Institute, Kaleida
Health, Buffalo, New York

BERNARD R. BENDOK, MD, MSCI
Department of Neurological Surgery, Precision
Neuro-therapeutics Innovation Lab,
Neurosurgery Simulation and Innovation Lab,

Department of Radiology, Department of
Otolaryngology, Mayo Clinic Hospital, Mayo
Clinic, Phoenix, Arizona

ARNAU BENET, MD
Department of Neurological Surgery, University
of California San Francisco, San Francisco,
California

SIGURD BERVEN, MD
Professor in Residence, Chief of Spine Service,
Department of Orthopaedic Surgery, UC San
Francisco, San Francisco, California

SARAH K.B. BICK, MD
Resident, Department of Neurosurgery,
Massachusetts General Hospital, Boston,
Massachusetts

ROBERT W. BINA, MD
Division of Neurosurgery, Banner University
Medical Center, Tucson, Arizona

PATRICK B. BOLTON, MD
Department of Anesthesia & Periop Med, Mayo
Clinic Hospital, Mayo Clinic, Phoenix, Arizona

JOHN F. BURKE, MD, PhD
Department of Neurological Surgery, University
of California, San Francisco, San Francisco,
California

JAN-KARL BURKHARDT, MD
Department of Neurological Surgery, University
of California San Francisco, San Francisco,
California

SERGIO CAVALHEIRO, MD, PhD
Chairman, Neurosurgery Department, Federal
University of São Paulo–UNIFESP, São Paulo,
São Paulo, Brazil

BRIAN W. CHONG, MD, FRCP(C)
Department of Neurological Surgery,
Department of Radiology, Mayo Clinic
Hospital, Mayo Clinic, Phoenix, Arizona

**MARCOS DEVANIR SILVA DA COSTA, MD,
MSc**
International Fellow, Department of Pediatric
Neurosurgery, Nationwide Children's Hospital,
Columbus, Ohio; Neurosurgeon, Neurosurgery
Department, Federal University of São Paulo–
UNIFESP, São Paulo, São Paulo, Brazil

JASON M. DAVIES, MD, PhD
Assistant Professor of Neurosurgery &
Bioinformatics, University at Buffalo, State
University of New York, Buffalo, New York

**BART M. DEMAERSCHALK, MD, MSc,
FRCP(C)**
Department of Neurology, Mayo Clinic
Hospital, Mayo Clinic, Phoenix, Arizona

SANJAY S. DHALL, MD
Department of Neurological Surgery, University
of California, San Francisco, San Francisco,
California

ANTHONY DiGIORGIO, DO
Department of Neurosurgery, UC San
Francisco, San Francisco, California

EMAD N. ESKANDAR, MD
Professor, Department of Neurosurgery,
Massachusetts General Hospital, Boston,
Massachusetts

VERNARD S. FENNELL, MD, MSc
Endovascular Neurosurgery Fellow,
Department of Neurosurgery, Jacobs School
of Medicine and Biomedical Sciences,
University at Buffalo, State University of New
York, Gates Vascular Institute, Kaleida Health,
Buffalo, New York

RICHARD G. FESSLER, MD, PhD
Department of Neurosurgery, Rush University
Medical Center, Chicago, Illinois

RICARDO B. FONTES, MD, PhD
Assistant Professor, Department of
Neurosurgery, Rush University Medical Center,
Chicago, Illinois

ZOHER GHOGAWALA, MD
Professor and Chairman, Department of
Neurosurgery, Alan and Jacqueline Stuart
Spine Research Center, Lahey Hospital and
Medical Center, Burlington, Massachusetts;
Department of Neurosurgery, Tufts University
School of Medicine, Boston, Massachusetts

AMAN GUPTA, MD
Department of Neurological Surgery, Precision
Neuro-therapeutics Innovation Lab,
Neurosurgery Simulation and Innovation Lab,
Mayo Clinic Hospital, Mayo Clinic, Phoenix,
Arizona

**R. JOHN HURLBERT, MD, PhD, FRCSC,
FACS**
Division of Neurosurgery, Banner University
Medical Center, Tucson, Arizona

STEVEN N. KALKANIS, MD
Chair, Department of Neurosurgery, Henry
Ford Hospital, Detroit, Michigan

CHANDAN KRISHNA, MD
Department of Neurological Surgery, Mayo
Clinic Hospital, Mayo Clinic, Phoenix, Arizona

MICHAEL T. LAWTON, MD
Department of Neurological Surgery, University
of California San Francisco, San Francisco,
California

IAN LEE, MD
Senior Staff Neurosurgical Oncology, Department of Neurosurgery, Henry Ford Hospital, Detroit, Michigan

JEFFREY LEONARD, MD
Chief, Pediatric Neurosurgery Department, Nationwide Children's Hospital, Columbus, Ohio

ELAD I. LEVY, MD, MBA, FACS, FAHA
Collaborator, Toshiba Stroke & Vascular Research Center, University at Buffalo, State University of New York, Professor & Chair of Neurosurgery and Professor of Radiology, Jacobs School of Medicine and Biomedical Sciences, University at Buffalo, State University of New York, Medical Director, Neuroendovascular Services, Gates Vascular Institute, Kaleida Health, Buffalo, New York

JONATHAN J. LIU, MD
Department of Neurosurgery, Stanford University School of Medicine, Stanford, California

MARK K. LYONS, MD
Department of Neurological Surgery, Mayo Clinic Hospital, Mayo Clinic, Phoenix, Arizona

JAMAL McCLENDON Jr, MD
Department of Neurological Surgery, Mayo Clinic Hospital, Mayo Clinic, Phoenix, Arizona

ANTONIO FERNANDES MORON, MD, PhD
Chairman of the Obstetrics Department, Hospital and Maternity Santa Joana, Federal University of São Paulo–UNIFESP, São Paulo, São Paulo, Brazil

SABAREESH K. NATARAJAN, MD, MS
Endovascular Neurosurgery Fellow, Department of Neurosurgery, Jacobs School of Medicine and Biomedical Sciences, University at Buffalo, State University of New York, Gates Vascular Institute, Kaleida Health, Buffalo, New York

IMRAN NOORANI, MB BChir, MRCS
Academic Clinical Fellow, Department of Neurological Surgery, Barrow Neurological Institute, Phoenix, Arizona; Department of Neurosurgery, Addenbrooke's Hospital, Cambridge, United Kingdom

NARESH PATEL, MD
Department of Neurological Surgery, Mayo Clinic Hospital, Mayo Clinic, Phoenix, Arizona

DAVID W. POLLY Jr, MD
Professor and Chief of Spine Surgery, Departments of Orthopaedic Surgery and Neurosurgery, University of Minnesota, Minneapolis, Minnesota

VIJAY M. RAVINDRA, MD, MSPH
Resident, Department of Neurosurgery, Clinical Neurosciences Center, University of Utah, Salt Lake City, Utah; Stuart Spine Fellow, Department of Neurosurgery, Alan and Jacqueline Stuart Spine Research Center, Lahey Hospital and Medical Center, Burlington, Massachusetts

ADAM M. ROBIN, MS, MD
Neurosurgical Oncology Fellow, Department of Neurosurgery, Memorial Sloan Kettering Cancer Center, New York, New York

NADER SANAI, MD
Professor, Department of Neurological Surgery, Barrow Neurological Institute, Phoenix, Arizona

MITHUN G. SATTUR, MD
Department of Neurological Surgery, Precision Neuro-therapeutics Innovation Lab, Neurosurgery Simulation and Innovation Lab, Mayo Clinic Hospital, Mayo Clinic, Phoenix, Arizona

AYAN SEN, MD
Department of Critical Care Medicine, Mayo Clinic Hospital, Mayo Clinic, Phoenix, Arizona

HAKEEM J. SHAKIR, MD
Endovascular Neurosurgery Fellow, Department of Neurosurgery, Jacobs School of Medicine and Biomedical Sciences, University at Buffalo, State University of New York, Gates Vascular Institute, Kaleida Health, Buffalo, New York

HUSSAIN SHALLWANI, MD
Endovascular Neurosurgery Fellow, Department of Neurosurgery, Jacobs School of Medicine and Biomedical Sciences, University at Buffalo, State University of New York, Gates Vascular Institute, Kaleida Health, Buffalo, New York

ADNAN H. SIDDIQUI, MD, PhD, FACS, FAHA, FAANS
Vice-Chairman & Professor of Neurosurgery and Director of Neuroendovascular Fellowship Program, Department of Neurosurgery, Jacobs School of Medicine and Biomedical Sciences, University at Buffalo, State University of New York, Director, Neurosurgical Stroke Service, Kaleida Health, Chief Medical Officer, The Jacobs Institute, Director, Toshiba Stroke & Vascular Research Center, University at Buffalo, State University of New York, Buffalo, New York

KENNETH V. SNYDER, MD, PhD
Assistant Professor of Neurosurgery, and Neurology, University at Buffalo, State University of New York, Buffalo, New York

GARY K. STEINBERG, MD, PhD
Professor and Chairman, Department of Neurosurgery, Stanford University School of Medicine, Stanford, California

KRISTIN SWANSON, PhD
Department of Neurological Surgery, Precision Neuro-therapeutics Innovation Lab, Mayo Clinic Hospital, Mayo Clinic, Phoenix, Arizona

RICHARD S. ZIMMERMAN, MD
Department of Neurological Surgery, Mayo Clinic Hospital, Mayo Clinic, Phoenix, Arizona

Contents

Preface: Current Controversies in Spinal and Cranial Surgery   xiii

Russell R. Lonser and Daniel K. Resnick

Spinal Surgery

The Sacroiliac Joint   301

David W. Polly Jr

> The sacroiliac joint moves 2.5°. It is innervated with nociceptive fibers. It is a common cause of low back pain (15%–30%). Degenerative changes occur, especially after lumbosacral fusion. When performed in series, physical examination maneuvers are diagnostic. Confirmatory image-guided injections can aid the diagnosis. In randomized clinical trials, surgical treatment in appropriately selected patients has been demonstrated to be statistically and clinically superior to nonsurgical management.

Sacroiliac Fusion: Another "Magic Bullet" Destined for Disrepute   313

Robert W. Bina and R. John Hurlbert

> Pain related to joint dysfunction can be treated with joint fusion; this is a long-standing principle of musculoskeletal surgery. However, pain arising from the sacroiliac (SI) joint is difficult to diagnose. Several implant devices are available that promote fusion by simply crossing the joint space. Evidence establishing outcomes is misleading because of vague diagnostic criteria, flawed methodology, bias, and limited follow-up. Because of nonstandardized indications and historically inferior reconstruction techniques, SI joint fusion should be considered unproven. The indications and procedure in their present form are unlikely to stand up to close scrutiny or weather the test of time.

Is There Still a Role for Interspinous Spacers in the Management of Neurogenic Claudication?   321

Vijay M. Ravindra and Zoher Ghogawala

> Lumbar spinal stenosis with neurogenic claudication is prevalent in the elderly population. Decompression for this condition is the operation most commonly used to treat older patients. Because of the risks associated with open decompression procedures, particularly in older patients with comorbidities, minimally invasive procedures with implantation of interspinous process devices have been developed. This article reviews the current role of interspinous spacers in the treatment of lumbar spinal stenosis with neurogenic claudication and discusses the body of literature surrounding this treatment alternative.

Bone Morphogenic Protein Use in Spinal Surgery   331

John F. Burke and Sanjay S. Dhall

> Bone morphogenic protein (BMP) provides excellent enhancement of fusion in many spinal surgeries. BMP should be a cautionary tale about the use of industry-sponsored research, perceived conflicts of interest, and holding the field of spinal surgery

to the highest academic scrutiny and ethical standards. In the case of BMP, not having a transparent base of literature as it was approved led to delays in allowing this superior technology to help patients.

Lumbar Radiculopathy in the Setting of Degenerative Scoliosis: MIS Decompression and Limited Correction are Better Options   335

Ricardo B. Fontes and Richard G. Fessler

Surgery for adult spinal deformity (ASD) has emerged as an efficient treatment alternative, but it is fraught with potential perioperative morbidity, incompletely mitigated by emerging minimally invasive surgical techniques. In mild-to-moderate ASD balanced in the sagittal plane, there are situations in which the counterintuitive simple decompression through a foraminotomy or laminectomy, or even a short-segment fusion may be an attractive treatment. This article presents a case example and the authors' treatment rationale and reviews the limited available literature supporting it.

The Case for Deformity Correction in the Management of Radiculopathy with Concurrent Spinal Deformity   341

Sigurd Berven and Anthony DiGiorgio

The management of adult deformity varies significantly. Options range from nonoperative care to limited decompression to decompression with limited or extensive fusion. The appropriate surgical management is the approach that optimizes the likelihood of improvement in health-related quality of life, while limiting risks of complications and costs. Decompression alone is unreliable in the setting of significant deformity contributing to radiculopathy. Decompression with limited fusion is most appropriate for patients with age-appropriate global alignment of the spine, and decompression with more extensive fusion is most appropriate for patients with progressive deformity or with global sagittal or coronal malalignment.

Cranial Surgery

Hemicraniectomy for Ischemic and Hemorrhagic Stroke: Facts and Controversies   349

Aman Gupta, Mithun G. Sattur, Rami James N. Aoun, Chandan Krishna, Patrick B. Bolton, Brian W. Chong, Bart M. Demaerschalk, Mark K. Lyons, Jamal McClendon Jr, Naresh Patel, Ayan Sen, Kristin Swanson, Richard S. Zimmerman, and Bernard R. Bendok

Malignant large artery stroke is associated with high mortality of 70% to 80% with best medical management. Decompressive craniectomy (DC) is a highly effective tool in reducing mortality. Convincing evidence has accumulated from several randomized trials, in addition to multiple retrospective studies, that demonstrate not only survival benefit but also improved functional outcome with DC in appropriately selected patients. This article explores in detail the evidence for DC, nuances regarding patient selection, and applicability of DC for supratentorial intracerebral hemorrhage and posterior fossa ischemic and hemorrhagic stroke.

Direct Versus Indirect Bypass for Moyamoya Disease   361

Jonathan J. Liu and Gary K. Steinberg

Moyamoya disease is a progressive occlusive vasculopathy that involves the supraclinoid internal carotid arteries and Circle of Willis, and results in the formation of collateral vessels at the skull base. The progressive nature of this disease leads to cerebral ischemia and sometimes intracerebral hemorrhage. The treatment of moya-moya disease is mainly surgical revascularization, using revascularization techniques that include direct, indirect, and combined strategies. Here we discuss the available options for revascularization as well as our opinions regarding the surgical management of patients with moyamoya disease.

Flow Diversion after Aneurysmal Subarachnoid Hemorrhage   375

Sabareesh K. Natarajan, Hussain Shallwani, Vernard S. Fennell, Jeffrey S. Beecher, Hakeem J. Shakir, Jason M. Davies, Kenneth V. Snyder, Adnan H. Siddiqui, and Elad I. Levy

Flow diversion after aneurysmal subarachnoid hemorrhage (SAH) is the last treatment option for aneurysm occlusion when other methods of aneurysm treatment cannot be used because of the need for dual antiplatelet therapy. The authors' general protocol for treatment selection after aneurysmal SAH is provided to share with readers our approach to securing the aneurysm before embarking flow diversion for primary treatment or delayed adjunctive treatment to primary coiling. The authors' experience with flow diversion after aneurysmal SAH, review of pertinent literature, and the future of flow diversion after aneurysmal SAH are discussed.

Management of Small Incidental Intracranial Aneurysms   389

Jan-Karl Burkhardt, Arnau Benet, and Michael T. Lawton

Advances in neuroimaging and its widespread use for screening have increased the diagnosis of unruptured intracranial aneurysms (UIAs), including small-sized UIAs. The clinical management of these small-sized UIAs requires a patient-specific judgment of the risk of aneurysm rupture, if not treated, versus the risk of complications from surgical or endovascular treatment. Experienced cerebrovascular teams recommend treating small UIAs in young patients or in patients with more than one aneurysm rupture risk factor who also have a reasonable life expectancy. However, individual overall assessment of risk is critical for patients with UIAs to decide the next steps of care.

Surgical Management of Incidental Gliomas   397

Imran Noorani and Nader Sanai

Detailed brain imaging studies discover gliomas incidentally before clinical symptoms or signs show. These tumors represent an early stage in the natural history of gliomas. Left untreated, they are likely to progress to a symptomatic stage and transform to malignant gliomas. A greater extent of resection delays the onset of malignant transformation and prolongs patient survival. Because incidental gliomas are typically smaller and less likely to be in eloquent brain locations, there is a strong case for early surgical intervention to maximize resection and improve outcomes. This article discusses developments in the surgical management of low-grade gliomas.

Reoperation for Recurrent Glioblastoma Multiforme   407

Adam M. Robin, Ian Lee, and Steven N. Kalkanis

The role of reoperation for glioblastoma multiforme (GBM) recurrence is currently unknown. However, multiple studies have indicated that survival and quality of life are improved with a repeat operation at the time of disease recurrence. Prognosis is likely interdependent on several factors, including age, functional status, initial resection status, disease location, and surgical efficacy. However, there are significant data indicating no survival benefit for reoperation. This comprehensive literature review considering the controversial question of whether to operate for progressive or recurrent GBM seeks to evaluate the current available evidence and report on its conclusions.

Surgical Treatment of Trigeminal Neuralgia   429

Sarah K.B. Bick and Emad N. Eskandar

Trigeminal neuralgia is characterized by severe, episodic pain in the trigeminal nerve distribution. Medical therapy is the first line treatment. For patients with refractory pain, a variety of procedures including microvascular decompression, percutaneous radiofrequency rhizotomy, percutaneous glycerol rhizotomy, percutaneous balloon compression, and stereotactic radiosurgery are available. We review the literature and suggest that microvascular decompression remains the gold standard operative therapy. For patients with recurrent pain or who are poor operative candidates, percutaneous radiofrequency rhizotomy offers the best pain response rates and has the advantage of being able to selectively target affected trigeminal divisions.

Comparison of Prenatal and Postnatal Management of Patients with Myelomeningocele   439

Sergio Cavalheiro, Marcos Devanir Silva da Costa, Antonio Fernandes Moron, and Jeffrey Leonard

Myelomeningocele (MMC) is a costly lifetime disease with many comorbidities, including sensory and motor lower limb disability, bladder/bowel dysfunction, scoliosis, club foot, and hydrocephalus. MMC treatment options have changed over time because routine use of fetal ultrasonography and MRI has provided prenatal diagnosis and the potential for fetal surgery. There is still no consensus on how to treat the MMC diagnoses prenatally, mainly related to the infrastructure required to operate on pregnant patients. This article provides an overview of prenatal and postnatal MMC repair and the features in the prenatal diagnosis.

Index   449

NEUROSURGERY CLINICS OF NORTH AMERICA

FORTHCOMING ISSUES

October 2017
Intraoperative Imaging
J. Bradley Elder and Ganesh Rao, *Editors*

January 2018
Cervical Myelopathy
Michael G. Fehlings and Junichi Mizuno,
Editors

RECENT ISSUES

April 2017
Subdural Hematomas
E. Sander Connolly Jr and Guy M. McKhann II,
Editors

January 2017
Adult and Pediatric Spine Trauma
Douglas L. Brockmeyer and Andrew T. Dailey,
Editors

Preface
Current Controversies in Spinal and Cranial Surgery

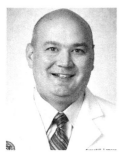 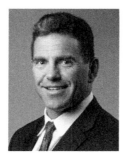

Russell R. Lonser, MD   Daniel K. Resnick, MD
Editors

This issue of the *Neurosurgery Clinics of North America* focuses on current controversies in spinal surgery and cranial surgery. Each of the spinal or cranial controversies is covered by international leaders in the field and contains state-of-the-art information. The purpose of this issue is to provide surgeons with readily available and concise, yet comprehensive, reviews of controversial topics to allow for best-informed decision-making and patient care.

Controversies in spinal surgery are nothing new. Rapid advances in medical technology have often outpaced rational deliberation of the indications and results of new procedures. Spine surgery has seen explosive growth in implantable technologies, as fixation techniques have gone from interspinous process wiring to segmental instrumentation techniques to interbody applications through a variety of portals. The causes of "back pain" treated by spine surgeons have expanded and now include degenerative deformity and the sacroiliac joint. With each technological advance, there is a predictable surge of enthusiasm followed by a period of uncertainty followed, in many cases, by disapproval. It is our responsibility to discuss the potential benefits and drawbacks of emerging technologies, as soon as evidence becomes available. We discuss the emerging technology of sacroiliac joint fusion, the potential rebirth of spinous process fixation, the use of bone morphogenetic protein, and the plusses and minuses of minimally invasive versus maximally corrective surgery for neurologic compromise associated with degenerative deformity.

Similarly, controversies over the management of intracranial pathology have existed since before the inception of neurologic surgery. New insights into the pathobiology of intracranial disease, deeper understanding (or lack thereof) of the natural history of various intracranial lesions, the limited number of large controlled patient studies that examine outcomes, and evolving technologies have been the foundation for these disputes. Here, we discuss the critical vascular controversies surrounding ischemia, including the role of hemicraniectomy for ischemic/hemorrhagic stroke and treatment strategies for moyamoya disease. We examine controversies in cerebral aneurysm management, including endovascular flow diversion after subarachnoid hemorrhage and the management of small incidental cerebrovascular aneurysms. We analyze controversies in surgical neurooncology, including reoperation for recurrent glioblastoma and the surgical management of incidental gliomas. We discuss the various surgical options for medically intractable trigeminal neuralgia. Finally, the management and outcomes for

Neurosurg Clin N Am 28 (2017) xiii–xiv
http://dx.doi.org/10.1016/j.nec.2017.04.001
1042-3680/17/© 2017 Published by Elsevier Inc.

neurosurgery.theclinics.com

prenatal versus postnatal management are defined for myelomeningocele patients.

Russell R. Lonser, MD
Department of Neurological Surgery
Ohio State University Wexner Medical Center
410 West 10th Avenue
N1047 Doan Hall
Columbus, OH 43210, USA

Daniel K. Resnick, MD
Department of Neurological Surgery
University of Wisconsin School of Medicine
600 Highland Avenue, Room K4/834
Madison, WI 53726, USA

E-mail addresses:
russell.lonser@osumc.edu (R.R. Lonser)
resnick@neurosurgery.wisc.edu (D.K. Resnick)

The Sacroiliac Joint

David W. Polly Jr, MD[a,b,*]

KEYWORDS

- Sacroiliac joint • SI joint • SIJ • Sacroiliac joint fusion • Low back pain

KEY POINTS

- The sacroiliac joint is a common cause of low back pain and should be included in the diagnosis.
- Nonoperative treatment of sacroiliac pain is expensive and surgical treatment is cost-effective in appropriately selected patients.
- High-quality clinical trials have demonstrated statistically and clinically significant improvement compared with nonsurgical management in appropriately selected patients.
- Spinal fusion to the sacrum increases degeneration of the sacroiliac joint.

The sacroiliac (SI) joint connects the spine to the pelvis and transmits the load of the body to the lower extremities (**Fig. 1**). It has a synovial portion and a large ligamentous area.[1] It has a unique pattern of motion called nutation counternutation (**Fig. 2**). The sacrum essentially flexes and extends. The iliac wings oscillate in the opposite direction to the sacrum. The normal motion is only 2.5°.[2,3] The surface of the joint is convoluted and provides a relatively large surface area for the volume of space it occupies. The SI joint is innervated.[4] The pattern of innervation is debated but can be from both dorsal and ventral. It has pain sensing nerve endings within the joint.[5]

Somewhere between 15% and 30% of low back pain may well arise from the SI joint.[6-9] The pattern of SI joint pain has significant overlap for spine-based pain and hip-based pain, making the differential diagnosis critical. It seems that some of the failures from low back pain surgery come from wrong diagnosis, such as a positive MRI finding that is actually asymptomatic.[10,11] Also with advances in hip arthroscopy, clinicians are beginning to understand more about pain generators within the hip. Unfortunately, imaging studies alone do not differentiate spine, hip, or SI pain. There can be abnormalities in any of the 3 areas but they may or may not be symptomatic.[12]

The diagnosis of the SI joint as a pain generator is based on physical examination of the SI joint and confirmatory diagnostic injection.[13,14] Similarly, the hip and spine need to be ruled out as pain generators. The physical examination maneuvers most commonly relied on for diagnosing the SI joint as a pain generator include flexion abduction external rotation (FABER) (**Fig. 3**), thigh thrust (**Fig. 4**), pelvic gapping (**Fig. 5**), pelvic compression (**Fig. 6**), and Gaenslen test (**Fig. 7**). If 3 of these are positive, then the pretest probability that a diagnostic injection will be positive is approximately 85%. Additional helpful physical examination findings are the Fortin finger test in which the patient points to the posterior superior iliac spine (PSIS) at the place where it hurts, tenderness to palpation over the PSIS, an ipsilateral positive Trendelenburg test (while standing on 1 leg the contralateral pelvis drops instead being able to be maintained horizontal), and pain over the PSIS with resisted supine active straight leg raise test.

Disclosures: There are no industry conflicts of interest. Dr Polly has been a clinical investigator in a clinical trial sponsored by SI-Bone but has not received any financial remuneration.
[a] Department of Orthopaedic Surgery, University of Minnesota, 2450 Riverside Avenue South, Minneapolis, MN 55454, USA; [b] Department of Neurosurgery, University of Minnesota, 420 Delaware Street SE, Minneapolis, MN 55455, USA
* Department of Orthopaedic Surgery, University of Minnesota, 2450 Riverside Avenue South, Minneapolis, MN 55454.
E-mail address: pollydw@umn.edu

Neurosurg Clin N Am 28 (2017) 301–312
http://dx.doi.org/10.1016/j.nec.2017.03.003
1042-3680/17/© 2017 Elsevier Inc. All rights reserved.

neurosurgery.theclinics.com

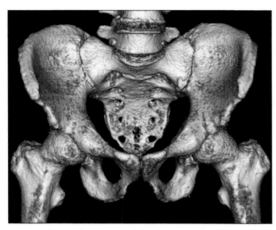

Fig. 1. Three-dimensional (3D) view of pelvis and SI joints.

Examination of the hip should include range of motion, especially internal rotation; femoral acetabular impingement testing; and a loaded grind or scour test. Palpation of the greater trochanter for tenderness is also crucial. Asking patients if it is their typical pain, as opposed to just asking if it is painful, helps to focus on their particular pain generator. Piriformis syndrome can present with symptoms in the same area. Spine examination typically involves formal neurologic testing of L4-S1, rotation plus extension, palpation for midline and facet tenderness, and palpation of the lateral border of the quadratus lumborum, looking for muscle spasm.

Plain radiographs are the starting point for imaging. A true anteroposterior (AP; Ferguson view) of the sacrum and a lateral of the pelvis are the best views for imaging the SI joint. In addition, an AP of the pelvis that includes the hips helps to rule out obvious hip osteoarthritis. An AP and

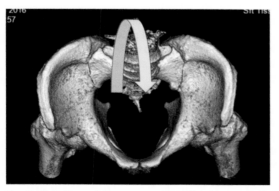

Fig. 2. Nutation of the sacrum. Nutation is essentially flexion of the sacrum (*arrow*) while counternutation is extension. The iliac wings are simultaneously counter-rotating.

lateral of the lumbar spine may point to obvious spinal pathologic conditions, such as spondylolisthesis or flatback syndrome with a pelvic incidence lumbar lordosis mismatch. The next step in imaging is probably an advanced axial imaging study of the pelvis and perhaps lower lumbar spine. This is primarily to rule out other unusual problems, such as tumors, infection, or stress fractures (**Fig. 8**). The final step is confirmatory diagnostic injection. This needs to be image-guided with contrast, demonstrating that the injection is into the intra-articular portion of the joint. If the injection is extra-articular or if it rapidly extravasates via an incompetent anterior joint capsule, interpretation of the pain response is very difficult. It is also useful to have the patients hold their pain medication and to do provoking activities before the injection. If the injection is equivocal or difficult to technically accomplish, then a computed tomography (CT)-guided injection can facilitate accessing the joint and ensuring that the injection is intra-articular. There is debate about what constitutes a positive response, but the best clinical trial data available suggest that a 50% response is predictive of patients who will respond to surgical management.[15] Having the patient do provoking activities after the injection is also very helpful to confirm or refute the joint as the pain generator. It is also common to need to inject the hip joint to rule it out as the pain generator. Ruling out the spine is more difficult. The role and benefit of intra-articular steroids in SI joint injections is less clear. The rate of usage of injections has markedly increased.[16]

Nonoperative management of the SI joint is commonly used but the response rate and durability are less clear. Physical therapy for a core stabilization type of approach can potentially be helpful. Manual therapy, be it administered by osteopathic or chiropractic techniques, can be helpful. The use of an SI belt can also be helpful. It is unclear what role medications play in terms of relief of pain. Certainly, for patients with a spondyloarthropathy, medications can make a significant difference. The last line of nonoperative management is radiofrequency ablation (RFA). There have been several trials looking at RFA.[17] The response rate and durability are variable, perhaps depending on the technique used (and the number of dorsal rami ablated), as well as the variability of the patient response.

SI joint pain can be profoundly debilitating. In terms of the burden of disease, it is as equally debilitating as hip and knee osteoarthritis that requires total joint arthroplasty, and spinal stenosis and spondylolisthesis that requires surgical management.[18,19]

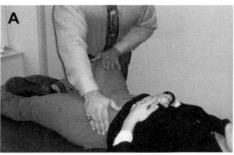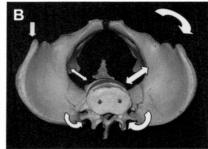

Fig. 3. Provocation test: (*A*) Patrick or FABER test. (*B*) 3D view with movement (*arrows*). ([*A*] *From* Sembrano JN, Reiley MA, Polly DW, et al. Diagnosis and treatment of sacroiliac joint pain. Curr Orthop Pract 2008;22(4):347; with permission.)

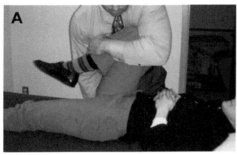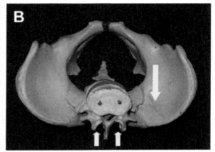

Fig. 4. Provocation test: (*A*) Thigh thrust, femoral shear, or posterior shear test. (*B*) 3D view with movement (*arrows*). ([*A*] *From* Sembrano JN, Reiley MA, Polly DW, et al. Diagnosis and treatment of sacroiliac joint pain. Curr Orthop Pract 2008;22(4):347; with permission.)

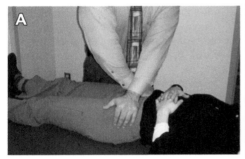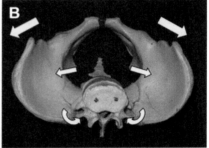

Fig. 5. Provocation test: (*A*) Distraction or pelvic gapping test. (*B*) 3D view with movement (*arrows*). ([*A*] *From* Sembrano JN, Reiley MA, Polly DW, et al. Diagnosis and treatment of sacroiliac joint pain. Curr Orthop Pract 2008;22(4):347; with permission.)

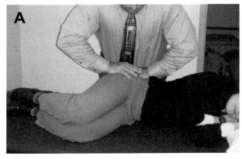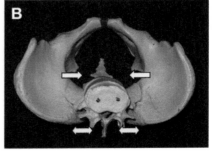

Fig. 6. Provocation test: (*A*) Pelvic compression or approximation test. (*B*) 3D view with movement (*arrows*). ([*A*] *From* Sembrano JN, Reiley MA, Polly DW, et al. Diagnosis and treatment of sacroiliac joint pain. Curr Orthop Pract 2008;22(4):347; with permission.)

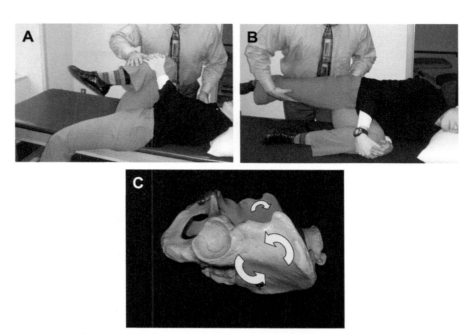

Fig. 7. Provocation test: Gaenslen or pelvic torsion test. Performed either (*A*) supine or (*B*) side lying. (*C*) 3D view with movement (*arrows*). ([*A, B*] *From* Sembrano JN, Reiley MA, Polly DW, et al. Diagnosis and treatment of sacroiliac joint pain. Curr Orthop Pract 2008;22(4):347; with permission.)

When nonoperative management has failed, surgery is a potential option. At least 17 different surgical techniques that have been described.[20] The original description was by Smith-Petersen.[21] Until recently, most literature was based on retrospective case series without prospectively collected patient-reported outcomes. Recently, there have been technological advances allowing

for minimally invasive techniques that have lessened the collateral damage associated with SI joint fusion. The use of minimally invasive techniques has significantly increased and the use of conventional open surgery has substantially declined (**Fig. 9**).[22]

The best studied technique, by far, has been the use of porous coated triangular titanium rods (iFuse Implant System, SI-BONE, Inc, San Jose, CA, USA) placed across the iliosacral joint. Comparing this technique with nonsurgical management, there have been 2 randomized controlled trials (RCTs),[23,24] 1 prospective cohort study,[25] 3 comparative effectiveness studies,[26–28] and numerous retrospective cohort studies.[26,27,29] Follow-up in 2 of the retrospective cohort studies has extended to 5 years.[30,31]

The surgical technique involves the transmuscular access to the outer table of the ilium; placing a Kirschner wire across the joint, either under fluoroscopic or image guidance; and drilling, broaching, and then press-fitting the implant. Typically, 3 implants are used (**Fig. 10**). In small pelves, sometimes only 2 can be placed. Safely placing these implants depends on a thorough understanding of sacropelvic anatomy and patient-specific anatomy. In approximately 5% of patients, there is a dysmorphic sacrum (or a transitional lumbosacral vertebra) that significantly alters the safe corridors for implant placement (**Fig. 11**).

Fig. 8. Imaging studies and pain. SI joint arthritic spurring shown on axial CT. An anterior osteophyte spanned the SI joint but the patient still had ipsilateral pain.

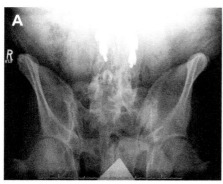
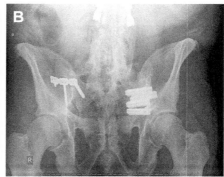

Fig. 9. Open and minimally invasive surgery. (*A*) This patient underwent a right-sided open anterior ilioinguinal approach fusion and plating. The left side was done minimally invasively. (*B*) Note the transitional lumbosacral vertebra.

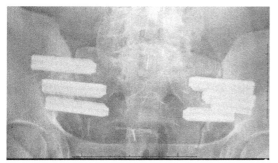

Fig. 10. SI joint fusion implants. Well-fixed right sided triangular titanium implants with left-sided halo formation on the left.

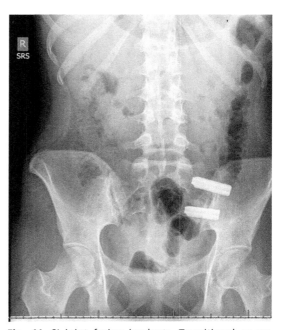

Fig. 11. SI joint fusion implants. Transitional or up-sloped sacrum with nonpermissive anatomy. Only 2 implants could be placed using intra-operative navigation.

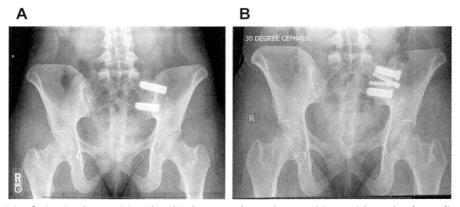

Fig. 12. SI joint fusion implant revision. (*A*, *B*) Subsequent loosening requiring revision using large diameter hollow screws and supplemental screw fixation.

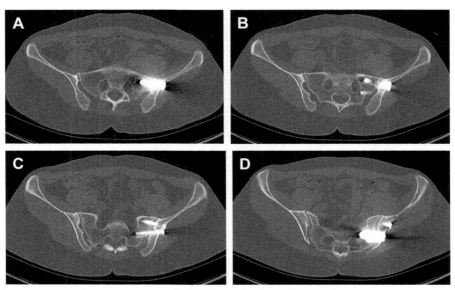

Fig. 13. SI joint fusion implant revision. (*A–D*) CT showing bridging bore cephalad.

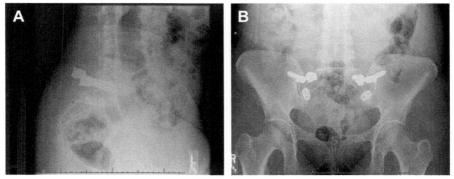

Fig. 14. SI joint fusion revision. (*A, B*) An alternative posterior technique of intra-articular cage placement with supplemental screw rod fixation.

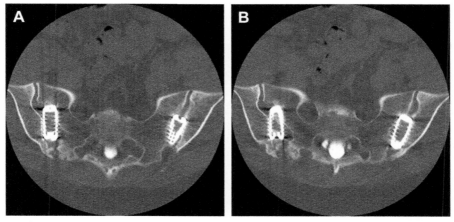

Fig. 15. SI joint fusion revision. (*A, B*) Right-sided cage placement has subsided into the sacrum, which has softer bone than the ilium.

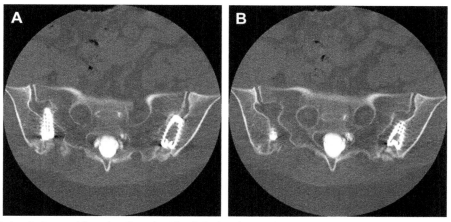

Fig. 16. SI joint fusion revision. (*A, B*) Both sides failed to have adequate bony healing.

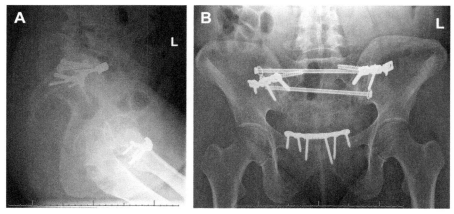

Fig. 17. SI joint fusion revision. (*A, B*) Cage removal, iliosacral screw fixation, and open anterior fusion were done after anterior symphysis pubis plating failed.

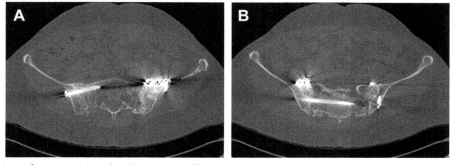

Fig. 18. SI joint fusion revision. (*A, B*) CT scans of bridging trabecular bone.

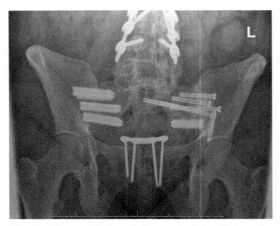

Fig. 19. Iliosacral fusion. Salvage of minimally invasive SI fusion. Anterior plating of the symphysis did not improve symptoms. The left side had implant removal, bone grafting through the defects, and iliosacral screw placement.

When using C-arm imaging, it is critical to be able to obtain good inlet, outlet, and lateral imaging. The outlet view insures avoidance of the neural foramina. The inlet view shows the spinal canal. The lateral view shows the anterior sacral border. The placement of the guidewire and the implant must be good on all 3 views. At the University of Minnesota, we have chosen to use intraoperative cone-beam CT and image guidance for implant placement. This has allowed a high degree of reliability of implant placement, even in cases of unusual anatomy. Because the sacral ala can have very vacuous cancellous bone, we have progressed to more frequent use of longer implants that, potentially, better engage sacral bone. We also routinely do postimplant placement check spins and have, on rare occasion (2 out of >450 implants, unpublished data, D.W. Polly, MD, 2010–2017), repositioned implants there were perhaps a little long.

A   B

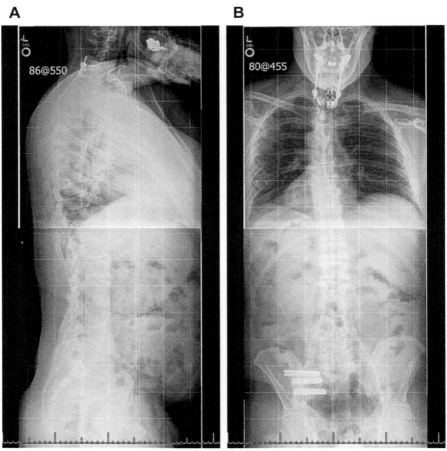

Fig. 20. Sagittal imbalance with SI joint pain. (*A*, *B*) This patient with sagittal imbalance had his SI joint fused uneventfully.

Postoperative management involves crutch ambulation touch weightbearing for 3 weeks. After this period, it is important to have the patients work with physical therapy because they will often have a significantly altered gait pattern. It is also common to see patients develop quadratus lumborum spasm during this time due to their altered gait. Prophylactically teaching the patients how to stretch out their quadratus lumborum has been helpful.

The inclusion criteria for the prospective studies have been consistent.[23–25] It has included 6 months of nonsurgical management in a stepwise fashion (including the use of RFA), at least 3 of 5 positive physical examination findings, and at least a 50% reduction in pain with an image-guided diagnostic injection. These studies show a remarkably consistent reduction in pain as measured by a visual analog scale (VAS) and Oswestry Disability Index. Minimum clinically important differences (MCIDs) in pain reduction were achieved in approximately 85% of patients in these trials in the surgical arm. Conversely, only approximately 20% of the nonsurgically managed (NSM) patients achieved a MCID and 80% of the NSM patients subsequently crossed over to surgical treatment after 6 months of continued failure of NSM. Complications rates were low. The published data on revision rates were on the order of 3%.[32] Unpublished data from the University of Minnesota showed revision rates to be approximately 7% in the first 2 years of experience, perhaps it is lower now. When failure occurs, it is from sacral side loosening (**Figs. 12** and **13**). The sacral bone is far less dense than the ilium (**Figs. 14–18**).[33]

Pooled patient level data from the 2 RCTs and the prospective cohort study are now in press.[34] With the larger numbers available, some risk factors for success and failure have been identified. In patients undergoing surgical treatment, slightly smaller responses were seen in smokers and opioid users, and slightly larger improvements were seen in those with longer pain durations and higher age. Overall, the surgical cohorts showed clinically meaningful improvement with VAS for pain reduced 38 points (on a 0–100 scale)

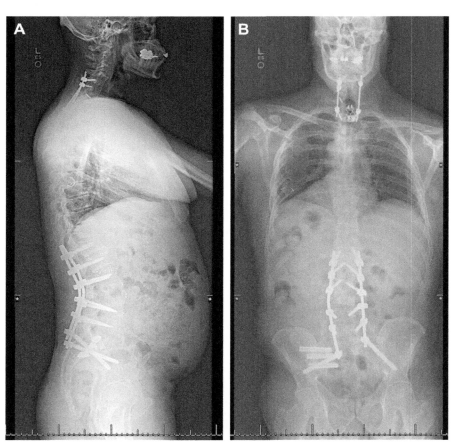

Fig. 21. Sagittal imbalance with SI joint pain. (*A, B*) Persistent pain following SI joint fusion requiring an osteotomy.

compared with nonsurgical cohorts. Oswestry Disability Index scores improved 18 points more than nonsurgical management. Improvement magnitude in VAS and ODI were consistent in the RCTs, the prospective cohort, and in many retrospective cohorts.[23,25,29]

There are several other techniques and devices available for fusing the SI joint. To date, there are limited published clinical data available (some small retrospective cohort series). It is unclear if these devices and techniques will be better, worse, or the same as porous coated triangular titanium rods.[35–38]

SI joint degeneration below spine fusions is becoming more recognized (**Fig. 19**). Ha and colleagues[39] studied this and found that in subjects with the spine fused to the sacrum, 75% developed radiographic degeneration within 5 years, whereas only 38% of patients with floating fusions developed radiographic degeneration. Bone graft harvesting of the outer table of the ilium probably also contributes to SI pain.[40] Inadvertent violation of the SI joint can often be evident on CT scans.[41]

This bone graft defect can also make implant placement technically more challenging.

Because clinicians are recognizing sagittal imbalance more often, it probably also plays a role in SI joint pain (**Figs. 20–22**). With sagittal imbalance, the posterior musculature must exert greater force to maintain upright posture. With the origin of fascia and musculature off of the ilium, this will exert greater force on the posterior pelvis. If a patient has positive sagittal balance and SI joint pain, fixing the sagittal imbalance first is probably the preferred way to go.

In long fusions to the sacrum, the use of pelvic fixation has increased. Conventional iliac screws used in a Galveston technique have a relatively high rate of being symptomatic. This instrumentation spans the SI joint in an extra-articular fashion. It is not uncommon to see a windshield-wiper effect or halo formation around these screws (see **Fig. 10**), indicating ongoing SI joint motion. More recently, S2 alar iliac fixation has been adopted.[42] This results in lower implant profile and less

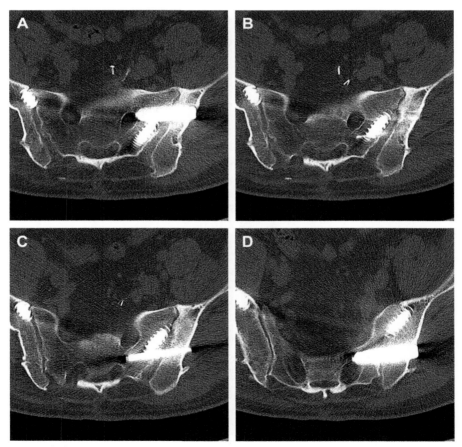

Fig. 22. Sagittal imbalance with SI joint pain. (*A–D*) Placing pelvic fixation around SI implants is technically challenging.

muscle dissection but directly violates and crosses the SI joint. It is unclear if this will decrease or increase the rate of SI joint pain in long fusion patients. The author's initial impression is that it seems less common but the exact reason is unclear. This is consistent with data reported by Ohtori and colleagues.[43] Experience from the pelvic trauma literature suggests that transsacral-transiliac screws crossing an uninjured SI joint do not significantly affect patient pain.[44]

In summary, the SI joint moves, is innervated, can be a pain generator, and can be reliably diagnosed and reliably treated with reasonably predictable good but not great results. Looking for it as a part of the differential diagnosis in patients with low back and buttock pain will increase the probability of successful treatment of this group of patients.

REFERENCES

1. Vleeming A, Schuenke MD, Masi AT, et al. The sacroiliac joint: an overview of its anatomy, function and potential clinical implications. J Anat 2012; 221(6):537–67.
2. Kibsgård TJ, Røise O, Sturesson B, et al. Radiosteriometric analysis of movement in the sacroiliac joint during a single-leg stance in patients with long-lasting pelvic girdle pain. Clin Biomech (Bristol, Avon) 2014;29(4):406–11.
3. Sturesson B, Uden A, Vleeming A. A radiostereometric analysis of movements of the sacroiliac joints during the standing hip flexion test. Spine (Phila Pa 1976) 2000;25(3):364–8.
4. Fortin JD, Kissling RO, O'Connor BL, et al. Sacroiliac joint innervation and pain. Am J Orthop (Belle Mead NJ) 1999;28(12):687–90.
5. Szadek KM, Hoogland PV, Zuurmond WW, et al. Nociceptive nerve fibers in the sacroiliac joint in humans. Reg Anesth Pain Med 2008;33(1): 36–43.
6. Bernard TN Jr, Kirkaldy-Willis WH. Recognizing specific characteristics of nonspecific low back pain. Clin Orthop Relat Res 1987;(217):266–80.
7. Maigne JY, Aivaliklis A, Pfefer F. Results of sacroiliac joint double block and value of sacroiliac pain provocation tests in 54 patients with low back pain. Spine (Phila Pa 1976) 1996;21(16):1889–92.
8. Schwarzer AC, Aprill CN, Bogduk N. The sacroiliac joint in chronic low back pain. Spine (Phila Pa 1976) 1995;20(1):31–7.
9. Sembrano JN, Polly DW Jr. How often is low back pain not coming from the back? Spine (Phila Pa 1976) 2009;34(1):E27–32.
10. Ackerman SJ, Polly DW Jr, Knight T, et al. Nonoperative care to manage sacroiliac joint disruption and degenerative sacroiliitis: high costs and medical resource utilization in the United States Medicare population. J Neurosurg Spine 2014;20(4):354–63.
11. Ackerman SJ, Polly DW Jr, Knight T, et al. Comparison of the costs of nonoperative care to minimally invasive surgery for sacroiliac joint disruption and degenerative sacroiliitis in a United States commercial payer population: potential economic implications of a new minimally invasive technology. Clinicoecon Outcomes Res 2014;6:283–96.
12. Morgan PM, Anderson AW, Swiontkowski MF. Symptomatic sacroiliac joint disease and radiographic evidence of femoroacetabular impingement. Hip Int 2013;23(2):212–7.
13. Kokmeyer DJ, Van der Wurff P, Aufdemkampe G, et al. The reliability of multitest regimens with sacroiliac pain provocation tests. J Manipulative Physiol Ther 2002;25(1):42–8.
14. Laslett M, Aprill CN, McDonald B, et al. Diagnosis of sacroiliac joint pain: validity of individual provocation tests and composites of tests. Man Ther 2005;10(3): 207–18.
15. Polly D, Cher D, Whang PG, et al, INSITE Study Group. Does level of response to SI joint block predict response to SI joint fusion? Int J Spine Surg 2016;10(4):1–13.
16. Manchikanti L, Hansen H, Pampati V, et al. Utilization and growth patterns of sacroiliac joint injections from 2000 to 2011 in the Medicare population. Pain Physician 2013;16(4):E379–90.
17. Cohen SP, Hurley RW, Buckenmaier CC 3rd, et al. Randomized placebo-controlled study evaluating lateral branch radiofrequency denervation for sacroiliac joint pain. Anesthesiology 2008;109(2):279–88.
18. Cher D, Polly D, Berven S. Sacroiliac joint pain: burden of disease. Med Devices (Auckl) 2014;7:73–81.
19. Cher DJ, Polly DW. Improvement in health state utility after sacroiliac joint fusion: comparison to normal populations. Global Spine J 2016;6(2):100–7.
20. Stark JG, Fuentes JA, Fuentes TI, et al. The history of sacroiliac joint arthrodesis: a critical review and introduction of a new technique. Curr Orthop Pract 2011;22(6):545–57.
21. Smith-Petersen M, Rogers W. End-result study of arthrodesis of the sacroiliac joint for arthritis—traumatic and nontraumatic. J Bone Joint Surg 1926;8: 118–36.
22. Lorio MP, Polly DW Jr, Ninkovic I, et al. Utilization of minimally invasive surgical approach for sacroiliac joint fusion in surgeon population of ISASS and SMISS membership. Open Orthop J 2014;8:1–6.
23. Polly DW, Swofford J, Whang PG, et al. Two-year outcomes from a randomized controlled trial of minimally invasive sacroiliac joint fusion vs. non-surgical management for sacroiliac joint dysfunction. Int J Spine Surg 2016;10(28):1–22.
24. Sturesson B, Kools D, Pflugmacher R, et al. Six-month outcomes from a randomized controlled trial

of minimally invasive SI joint fusion with triangular titanium implants vs conservative management. Eur Spine J 2017;26(3):708–19.

25. Duhon BS, Bitan F, Lockstadt H, et al. Triangular titanium implants for minimally invasive sacroiliac joint fusion: 2-year follow-up from a prospective multicenter trial. Int J Spine Surg 2016;10(13):1–27.

26. Ledonio CG, Polly DW Jr, Swiontkowski MF. Minimally invasive versus open sacroiliac joint fusion: are they similarly safe and effective? Clin Orthop Relat Res 2014;472(6):1831–8.

27. Ledonio CG, Polly DW Jr, Swiontkowski MF, et al. Comparative effectiveness of open versus minimally invasive sacroiliac joint fusion. Med Devices (Auckl) 2014;7:187–93.

28. Smith AG, Capobianco R, Cher D, et al. Open versus minimally invasive sacroiliac joint fusion: a multi-center comparison of perioperative measures and clinical outcomes. Ann Surg Innov Res 2013; 7(1):14.

29. Heiney J, Capobianco R, Cher D. A systematic review of minimally invasive sacroiliac joint fusion utilizing a lateral transarticular technique. Int J Spine Surg 2015;9(40):1–16.

30. Rudolf L, Capobianco R. Five-year clinical and radiographic outcomes after minimally invasive sacroiliac joint fusion using triangular implants. Open Orthop J 2014;8:375–83.

31. Vanaclocha V, Verdú-López F, Sánchez-Pardo M, et al. Minimally invasive sacroiliac joint arthrodesis: experience in a prospective series with 24 patients. J Spine 2014;3(5).

32. Miller LE, Reckling WC, Block JE. Analysis of post-market complaints database for the iFuse SI Joint Fusion System(R): a minimally invasive treatment for degenerative sacroiliitis and sacroiliac joint disruption. Med Devices (Auckl) 2013;6:77–84.

33. Hoel RJ, Ledonio CG, Takahashi T, et al. Sacral bone mineral density (BMD) assessment using opportunistic CT scans. J Orthop Res 2017;35(1):160–6.

34. Dengler J, Polly DW, Whang P, et al. Predictors of outcome in conservative and minimally invasive surgical management of pain originating from the sacroiliac joint – a pooled analysis. Spine J 2017. [Epub ahead of print].

35. Beck CE, Jacobson S, Thomasson E. A retrospective outcomes study of 20 sacroiliac joint fusion patients. Cureus 2015;7(4):e260.

36. Kube RA, Muir JM. Sacroiliac joint fusion: one year clinical and radiographic results following minimally invasive sacroiliac joint fusion surgery. Open Orthop J 2016;10:679–89.

37. Miller LE, Block JE. Minimally invasive arthrodesis for chronic sacroiliac joint dysfunction using the SImmetry SI Joint Fusion system. Med Devices (Auckl) 2014;7:125–30.

38. Rappoport LH, Luna IY, Joshua G. Minimally invasive sacroiliac joint fusion using a novel hydroxyapatite-coated screw: preliminary 1-year clinical and radiographic results of a 2-year prospective study. World Neurosurg 2017;101:493–7.

39. Ha K-Y, Lee J-S, Kim K-W. Degeneration of sacroiliac joint after instrumented lumbar or lumbosacral fusion: a prospective cohort study over five-year follow-up. Spine (Phila Pa 1976) 2008;33(11):1192–8.

40. Ebraheim NA, Elgafy H, Semaan HB. Computed tomographic findings in patients with persistent sacroiliac pain after posterior iliac graft harvesting. Spine (Phila Pa 1976) 2000;25(16):2047–51.

41. Dhawan A, Kuklo TR, Polly DW Jr. Analysis of iliac crest bone grafting process measures. Am J Orthop (Belle Mead NJ) 2006;35(7):322–6.

42. O'Brien JR, Yu WD, Bhatnagar R, et al. An anatomic study of the S2 iliac technique for lumbopelvic screw placement. Spine (Phila Pa 1976) 2009;34(12): E439–42.

43. Ohtori S, Sainoh T, Takaso M, et al. Clinical incidence of sacroiliac joint arthritis and pain after sacropelvic fixation for spinal deformity. Yonsei Med J 2012;53(2):416–21.

44. Heydemann J, Hartline B, Gibson ME, et al. Do transsacral-transiliac screws across uninjured sacroiliac joints affect pain and functional outcomes in trauma patients? Clin Orthop Relat Res 2016; 474(6):1417–21.

Sacroiliac Fusion
Another "Magic Bullet" Destined for Disrepute

 CrossMark

Robert W. Bina, MD, R. John Hurlbert, MD, PhD, FRCSC*

KEYWORDS

- Back pain • Spinal fusion • Evidence • Quackery

KEY POINTS

- The sacroiliac (SI) joints are load-bearing synovial-lined joints that can be affected by degenerative change and therefore in some circumstances MAY cause local pain.
- Diagnosis of painful SI joints has NOT been standardized and at the current time is best represented by (1) local pain at the sacral ala, (2) degenerative changes on imaging studies, AND (3) temporary relief from intra-articular injection of topical anesthetic agents and/or steroids.
- Current technology for SI joint fusion mimics first-generation stand-alone lumbar cages, promoting fusion simply by breaching the joint space.
- Evidence of benefit from SI fusion is poor because of imprecise diagnoses, flawed methodology, bias, and limited follow-up.
- SI fusion should be undertaken only with full disclosure to the patient that the indications and long-term results for the technique remain unproven.

INTRODUCTION

The diagnosis and treatment of low back pain is a complex process. Anatomic components are varied and numerous: bones, discs, ligaments, synovium, joints. Their interactions are even more complex.[1,2] Part and parcel with these moving pieces are complicated biomechanics in which changes in one part of the system affect other parts in clinically relevant ways. This article discusses sacroiliac joint dysfunction, its clinical impact, diagnosis, and nonoperative and operative treatments with a critical appraisal of a growing trend toward SI fusion.

EPIDEMIOLOGY

Low back pain is a common complaint in health care. In 1998 it is estimated that $26.3 billion was spent investigating and treating this complaint in the United States alone,[3] more than tripling in 2008 to $86 billion.[4,5] This dramatic cost escalation has been largely attributed to a significant increase in the number of patients seeking treatment for their low back pain symptoms over that 10-year period. In the current climate of value-based disease treatment, cost has become pivotal to health care policy. The 5-year cost to Medicare, our US federally funded health care system, specifically for treating SI joint dysfunction has already been appraised at $270 million.[6]

In any given year, the prevalence of low back pain in the adult community is estimated to range from 1.5% to 36.0%.[2] An individual's lifetime risk of suffering low back pain in adulthood severe enough to warrant medical consultation is 80% to 85%.[2,7–9] The vast majority of these episodes are self-limited, with 12-month remission rates of 54% to 90%.[2] The heterogeneity of these data are due to varied inclusion criteria and diverse mechanisms used to identify affected individuals, making them difficult to interpret.

Division of Neurosurgery, Banner University Medical Center, 1501 N Campbell Ave, Rm 4303, Tucson, AZ 85724, USA
* Corresponding author.
E-mail address: rjhurlbert@surgery.arizona.edu

Neurosurg Clin N Am 28 (2017) 313–320
http://dx.doi.org/10.1016/j.nec.2017.02.001
1042-3680/17/© 2017 Elsevier Inc. All rights reserved.

To effectively treat low back pain, accurate diagnoses and multidisciplinary expertise is necessary. Because of multiple etiologies and interactions, clinical history and examination remain fundamental to providing good outcomes. As an important anatomic structure in lumbo-sacral geography, sacroiliac joint dysfunction deserves at least passing consideration. Differentiation of low back pain from radicular pain is the first branch-point in the diagnostic algorithm.[8] The identification and treatment of nerve-root–mediated discomfort is reasonably objective and structured. Outcomes are predictable. However, the other causes of back pain exist in a twilight zone of low resolution and high noise. Only careful attention to the finer signs and symptoms helps the clinician avoid random diagnoses at the patient's expense. Location (midline or paraspinal), temporal profile, aggravating and relieving circumstances, provocative maneuvers based on anatomic substrates (eg, FABER, flexion vs extension), and psychological overlay (Waddell signs) are the primary tools available to clinicians helping to guide them through the quicksand of misguided intervention.

In those seeking treatment for low back pain, estimates of SI joint involvement range as high as 10% to 30%,[7,10–12] more frequently associated in patients with prior lumbar fusion.[13,14] However, calculating the true prevalence of SI joint dysfunction as the cause of low back pain is rife with difficulty as there are no "gold standard" criteria by which to make the diagnosis. Even the largest prevalence study relied only on clinical findings to establish the diagnosis.[15] This 1987 study of 1293 patients with low back pain from one clinician's practice is of limited utility: the report does not detail the specific manner of diagnosis and it reports a referred pain pattern as descriptive and therefore diagnostic. Of the 336 (23%) patients with "SI joint syndrome," only 66 (5%) were treated with joint injection yielding an amazing good-to-excellent response rate of 95%. Specious diagnostic criteria, selective intervention, and the retrospective nature of this study make its utility questionable.

Other prevalence studies suffer from even smaller sample sizes; for example, 43 patients from a selected low back pain population yielding 7 with SI joint-mediated pain (16% prevalence)[16] and 54 patients of whom 10 responded adequately to the diagnostic interventional treatment (18.5% prevalence).[17] Two smaller studies made use of interventional diagnostic criteria, yielding prevalence estimates of 16% to 30%.[10,15–17] However, these data are again from highly selected, nongeneralizable low back pain populations. The sum total of these studies further confounds the true prevalence of the disease because of inconsistent inclusion criteria, loose radiographic definitions, nonspecific clinical findings, and varied interventional techniques. Consequently, the true prevalence of SI-related low back pain is unknown.

ANATOMY

The sacroiliac joints are the largest axial joints in the body connecting the sacrum (and hence the spine) to the ilium of the pelvis. They are diarthrodial, planar, synovial joints lined by hyaline cartilage. As "joints" they are relatively immobile, reciprocally transmitting forces from the upper body to the lower extremities and vice versa (**Fig. 1**). Motion through these diarthroses is limited by the complex topography of the articular surfaces and by the multitude of strong, adjacent ligaments, including short and long dorsal sacroiliac ligaments, sacrotuberal, sacrospinous, iliolumbar, and interosseous ligaments. These ligaments connect the sacrum and the lumbar spine, dispersing forces and constraining motion, normal or dysfunctional, in the pelvis to the lumbar spine and vice versa.[18] Many of the pelvic muscles are also connected to the joints such as gluteus maximus, biceps femoris, and piriformis also affecting joint mobility and function.[10]

Motion in the sacroiliac joint is limited mainly to rotation around the S2 axis, more specifically called nutation and counter-nutation because of the sinusoidal rather than spherical pattern.[18] A number of studies have measured this motion, making use of a variety of motion-capture and video techniques. The most reliable studies have been performed in cadavers, and demonstrate excursion limited to 2.5° (0.8–3.9°) of rotation and 1.6 mm of translation.[19–21]

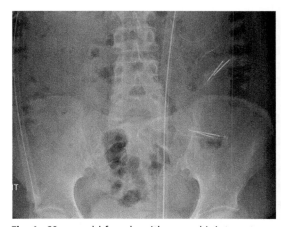

Fig. 1. 60 year old female with normal joint anatomy. This patient had no complaints of back or hip pain. Compare the anatomy in both of this patient's left and right SI joints with **Figs. 2** and **3**. (*Courtesy of* Jennifer Becker, Tucson, Arizona.)

Cadaveric studies have also indicated innervation of the SI joint to arise from dorsal and ventral rami of the L5 through S4 nerve roots,[22] supplying the articular surfaces with both unmyelinated and myelinated fibers (A-delta and C).[23,24]

POTENTIAL CAUSES OF SACROILIAC JOINT PAIN

Senescent changes in the joint can become apparent as early as puberty. These changes accumulate over a normal life span. Motion restriction becomes apparent in the 60s and more pervasive erosive changes in the 80s[10] (**Fig. 2**). Studies available to date suggest approximately half of patients with symptomatic SI joint dysfunction report an inciting history of trauma, commonly a combination of axial loading and rotation.[15,25] Cumulative wear and tear is proposed to account for patients unable to pinpoint a specific cause associated with their symptoms.[19,25] Other potential but rare causes proposed for SI joint degeneration and pain include pregnancy-associated ligamentous laxity with joint hypermobility,

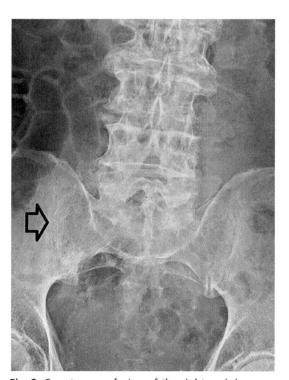

Fig. 2. Spontaneous fusion of the right and degeneration of the left SI joints in an 87-year-old man. The fused right joint is marked with an arrow. This patient had no pain complaints and was released from clinic. Compare the left SI joint in this patient with the left SI joint in the patient presented in **Fig. 3**. (*Courtesy of Jennifer Becker, MD.*)

sacroiliitis associated with ankylosing spondylitis, infection, enthesis injury or enthesopathy, sprain or strain, lumbar fusion and hip arthrodesis, stress and insufficiency fractures, metabolic causes (eg, gout, hyperparathyroidism), and tumors.[19]

DIAGNOSIS

Despite inherent limitations, clinical history has been the mainstay for diagnosing SI joint dysfunction. Symptoms suggesting SI-mediated pain are primarily identified as buttock pain and low back pain, reportedly present in 70% to 95% of patients with SI joint pathology.[26] However, as presenting symptoms, these complaints are clearly nonspecific and are at least as likely to indicate pain generators outside of the SI joints. To add to confusion, other studies report patients with SI joint dysfunction may deny lumbar discomfort at all.[27] Pain from SI joint dysfunction has been described to radiate into the thigh, groin, knee, and in some opinions even the lower leg.[8,26] However, not only are these symptoms nonspecific but they are more frequently encountered with pathology in and around the hip region. SI joint pain has also been proposed to be affected by changes in position; for example, sitting to standing, and to be frequently unilateral.[27] However, if one takes time to critically appraise these reports, they quickly realize there are no pathognomonic features pointing conclusively to the SI joint as the pain generator.

A variety of diagnostic clinical maneuvers elicited by physical examination have been proposed, summarized in **Table 1**.[8,18] Coexistence of at least 3 of these clinical signs are proposed

Table 1 Physical examination maneuvers for the clinical evaluation of sacroiliac joint pain	
Maneuver	**Motion**
Distraction	Pressure on anterior superior iliac crest
FABER (Patrick)	Flexion, abduction, external rotation of the thigh/hip
Gaenslen	Hip hyperextension
Thigh thrust	Adduction of flexed affected hip
Gillet	Standing thigh flexion
Compression	Compression of the thigh from lateral position
Fortin finger	Patient places 1 finger on source of pain 2 times

Sensitivity and specificity ranges from 78% to 79% and 85% to 94%, respectively, with 3 or more tests reproducing pain.

to confirm the SI joint as the primary source of low back pain,[8,27] claiming sensitivity near 80% and specificity in the range of 85% to 95%. However, as is so typical in SI pain literature, the discerning clinician will recognize these signs to be nonspecific and indeed far more synonymous with degenerative hip disease. Not surprisingly, the role of imaging in establishing a diagnosis of SI joint pain has so far been unproven[7] (see **Fig. 1**; **Fig. 3**).

Perhaps the most inherently compelling diagnostic criteria one would expect useful in making the diagnosis of SI pain is intra-articular injection. As with discography, this procedure can be undertaken to either provoke or abolish local pain symptoms. Joint capsular distension achieved through (for example) injection of saline may help confirm local pain generators. Local anesthesia achieved through infusion of topical agents (eg, bupivacaine hydrochloride [Marcaine]) may also be diagnostic and when combined with steroids perhaps therapeutic. Longer-term pain relief has been reported in some patients when injection is combined with rehabilitative therapy.[23] Unfortunately, evidence for this procedure as a diagnostic gold standard is moderate at best,[7] obtained from poorly randomized trials or limited comparative studies using concurrent or historical controls.

At the present time, the most compelling indicator of SI joint pain can only be proposed as focal discomfort localized primarily to the sacral ala, similar in characteristic to joint-associated pain

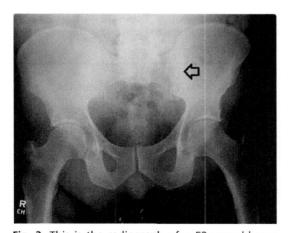

Fig. 3. This is the radiograph of a 52-year-old man diagnosed with left sacroiliitis. He had positive clinical findings of tenderness to palpation over the left SI joint, which is marked with an arrow. When compared with the normal radiograph seen in **Fig. 1**, the radiographic distinction is difficult to ascertain, but this film is distinctly different than the one presented in **Fig. 2**. This patient went on to have computed tomography–guided left SI joint injection. (*Courtesy of* Jennifer Becker, MD.)

recognized in every other part of the human body.[28] Caution, reservation, and even skepticism should be exercised on the part of the surgeon attempting to diagnose (let alone treat) this condition.

TREATMENT

It is very difficult to validate a treatment for a disease that cannot be reliably diagnosed. Not surprisingly then, therapeutic options are varied, poorly objectified, and remain within the same twilight zone as the treatment of lumbar facet pain. As discussed previously, intra-articular injection can be therapeutic. SI nerve ablation has been demonstrated to have some success most commonly through radiofrequency techniques, although cryotherapy[29] and sclerotic prolotherapy have also been reported.

Two randomized, placebo-controlled trials investigated the utility of radiofrequency ablation for the treatment of apparent SI joint pain.[30,31] The first of these[30] was composed of 28 patients with physical examination–evoked SI joint tenderness, long-term pain relief with prior steroid injection, and pain relief lasting longer than 6 hours after a diagnostic SI joint injection. In the treatment group, 57% of patients had relief at 6 months. However, this decreased to 14% (n = 2) at 1 year. None of the placebo group had pain relief at 3 months. Of the 11 patients who crossed over, only 4 (36%) had pain relief at 6 months. Interestingly, the investigators made use of a treatment technique NOT targeted specifically at the SI joints but instead directed toward the S1-S3 foramina.

The second study[31] was a prospective double-blind trial (2:1 treatment:control), but randomized only 51 patients. Inclusion was limited to patients with axial back pain lasting longer than 6 months and failure to improve with nonoperative treatment and other reasonable diagnoses excluded. Diagnosis was then confirmed with fluoroscopically guided intra-articular SI injection of local anesthetic producing pain relief for at least 4 hours and up to 7 days postinjection. Ablation was targeted in a similar fashion to the previously described study, at the foramina of S1-S3. At 3 months, 47% (n = 16) of treated patients improved, whereas 12% (n = 2) of control patients had continued relief. At 1 year, 9 of the initial treatment group had dropped out of the study, but of the remaining 25, 67% (n = 17) had symptomatic improvement. Sixteen of the control patients crossed over 3 months after randomization and 44% (n = 7) had significant pain relief that persisted into 6 months posttreatment. Together, these trials provide weak evidence that radiofrequency ablation directed at the root foramen of S1-S3 may reduce low back pain. However, they do little to further objectify the identification or treatment of SI-related pain.

Painter[32] first described a posterior surgical approach to the SI joint in 1908 using a long posterior incision and extensive soft tissue dissection for the treatment of a tuberculous joint and a traumatic fracture. The technique was later criticized by Smith-Petersen[33] in 1921 who instead championed a lateral approach to the joint through a bone window cut in the ilium, removal of cartilage and cortical bone, and fusion through iliac graft and screw fixation. The Painter[32] technique exposes the SI joint thoroughly, whereas the Smith-Petersen[33] approach exposes only a portion. More recently, the traditional Smith-Petersen[33] approach has fallen out of favor because of high nonunion rates, long inpatient stays, protracted recovery times, and poor clinical results prompting the development of minimally invasive approaches.[34–38] Modeled after Smith-Petersen,[33] the newer minimally invasive surgery (MIS) technique includes a lateral approach to the joint through a 3-cm incision, blunt fascial and muscular dissection to the level of the ilium, and fluoroscopically guided placement of a pin through the iliac portion of the SI joint into the sacral portion. Triangular plasma-coated titanium implants are then placed in the joint.[39]

Other described techniques of fixation include the following: a posterior approach using Cloward type bone plugs performed in 5 patients with apparently complete relief of symptoms[36]; a posterior percutaneous approach using bone morphogenetic protein–filled metal cages described in 13 patients with reported postoperative pain reduction[40]; a posterior midline approach with pedicle screw instrumentation[34]; and an anterior, open SI joint and pubic symphysis fusion performed in 7 patients claiming significant pain reduction scores with 1 year follow-up.[41]

Since 1998, a glut of studies have been published detailing indications, outcomes, and techniques for minimally invasive and percutaneous approaches to the SI joint, most claiming excellent clinical results. Many have been sponsored by device manufacturers competing for their spot in this new market. Rudolf[39] reported a series in which pain scores improved in 70% to 85% of patients within 1 year of surgery. However, lifting and bending ability was not significantly impacted. There were 10 perioperative complications (20%): 3 superficial skin infections; 1 deep infection; 2 hematomas; 2 new

sacral radiculopathies caused by implant migration; 1 malpositioned implant secondary to transitional lumbosacral anatomy; and 1 fracture. In this retrospective study, 91% of patients were satisfied with the surgery and the results. Another retrospective series of 20 patients treated with a single titanium cage filled with recombinant bone morphogenetic protein inserted through a posterior approach reported a successful fusion rate of 96.6% with 76.0% of patients reporting satisfaction with the operative outcome.[42]

To date, the best evidence in support of SI joint fusion is a multicenter trial in which 148 patients diagnosed with SI joint pain were randomized into 1 of 2 groups: surgery versus no surgery.[37,43] Surgical intervention consisted of the aforementioned MIS approach and implantation of a proprietary fixation system. At 6 months, 81.4% of the surgical group had successful treatment considered to be reduction in baseline pain, no reintervention, absence of surgical complication, and absence of new radicular symptoms. In the nonoperative group, success was simply considered as reduction in pain. Success in this group was 26.1% at 6 months. Patients were considered failures of nonsurgical management if they crossed over into the surgical group.[37] A report of these patients at 24 months was also published demonstrating stable pain reduction in the surgical group with 83% of patients reporting improvement.[43] This study was funded by SI-BONE (San Diego, California), incorporated, manufacturer of the implant grafts. Although presented as a randomized controlled trial of patients who had failed medical management, that all patients had failed medical management and that crossover was essentially guaranteed in the nonsurgical group, this trial is a case control trial. Three of the 4 primary outcomes reported in this trial were safety outcomes; only 1 reported clinical efficacy, which was a reduction in visual analogue scale (VAS) of at least 20 mm; the other 3 were absence of device-related adverse events, absence of device-related neurologic deficit, and absence of reintervention of SI joint pain. Most importantly, the inclusion criteria for this trial are a source of difficulty. As discussed previously, the clinical maneuvers used in this study are not specific.

There were no specific inclusion criteria for structural pathology; all inclusion criteria were clinical in nature hinging on a response to intra-articular injection after 30 to 60 minutes. The 2 radioablation trials discussed previously required a response lasting at least 4 to 6 hours for inclusion.

Not every study has published positive outcomes. In the series of 17 patients described by

Schutz and Grob[44] in which bilateral SI joint fusion was performed, 18% reported improvement in their pain, whereas 82% reported marked or severe pain at last follow-up. This study reported a nonunion rate of 41% with only a 35% incidence of radiographic union. The investigators cite difficulties in patient selection and question surgical technique in explaining these poor outcomes.

The only in vitro cadaveric study of laterally implanted, triangular, MIS sacroiliac implants has demonstrated that fixation techniques can significantly reduce artificially induced instability in flexion extension of the SI joint. However, they do not significantly reduce lateral bending or axial rotation movements.[45] This is not a minor limitation and is reminiscent of the biomechanical deficiencies of stand-alone lumbar cages popularized in the late 1990s.[46–48] Ultimately these suboptimal stabilization characteristics led to poor radiographic outcomes and complicated revisions.[49–53] Subsequently the technique was abandoned.

SUMMARY

In summary, pain related to joint dysfunction can be treated with joint fusion; this is a long-standing principle of musculoskeletal surgery. However, pain arising from the SI joint is difficult to diagnose. As of yet, there is no established algorithm of signs, symptoms, and investigations specific to this condition. Combined with a careful history, physical examination, and imaging studies, fluoroscopically guided SI joint injections may help to establish a diagnosis and predict benefit from surgical intervention. Surgical approaches vary: anterior, posterior, and lateral. Several implant devices are available on the market. In general, they promote fusion by simply crossing the joint space, similar to obsolete first-generation stand-alone lumbar cages. At the present time, evidence establishing short-term and long-term outcomes is misleading because of vague diagnostic criteria, flawed methodology, bias, and limited follow-up. Because of nonstandardized indications and historically inferior reconstruction techniques, SI joint fusion should be considered unproven. The indications and procedure in their present form are unlikely to stand up to close scrutiny or weather the test of time.

ACKNOWLEDGMENTS

Special thanks to Jennifer Becker, MD, for providing radiographic images.

REFERENCES

1. Hollingworth W, Todd CJ, King H, et al. Primary care referrals for lumbar spine radiography: diagnostic yield and clinical guidelines. Br J Gen Pract 2002; 52:475–80.
2. Hoy D, Brooks P, Blyth F, et al. The epidemiology of low back pain. Best Pract Res Clin Rheumatol 2010; 24:769–81.
3. Luo X, Pietrobon R, Sun SX, et al. Estimates and patterns of direct health care expenditures among individuals with back pain in the United States. Spine (Phila Pa 1976) 2004;29:79–86.
4. Ivanova JI, Birnbaum HG, Schiller M, et al. Real-world practice patterns, health-care utilization, and costs in patients with low back pain: the long road to guideline-concordant care. Spine J 2011;11: 622–32.
5. Kosloff TM, Elton D, Shulman SA, et al. Conservative spine care: opportunities to improve the quality and value of care. Popul Health Manag 2013;16: 390–6.
6. Ackerman SJ, Polly DW Jr, Knight T, et al. Nonoperative care to manage sacroiliac joint disruption and degenerative sacroiliitis: high costs and medical resource utilization in the United States Medicare population. J Neurosurg Spine 2014;20:354–63.
7. Boswell MV, Shah RV, Everett CR, et al. Interventional techniques in the management of chronic spinal pain: evidence-based practice guidelines. Pain Physician 2005;8:1–47.
8. Hooten WM, Cohen SP. Evaluation and treatment of low back pain: a clinically focused review for primary care specialists. Mayo Clin Proc 2015;90:1699–718.
9. Murray CJ, Atkinson C, Bhalla K, et al. The state of US health, 1990-2010: burden of diseases, injuries, and risk factors. JAMA 2013;310:591–608.
10. Cohen SP. Sacroiliac joint pain: a comprehensive review of anatomy, diagnosis, and treatment. Anesth Analg 2005;101:1440–53.
11. Sembrano JN, Polly DW Jr. How often is low back pain not coming from the back? Spine (Phila Pa 1976) 2009;34:E27–32.
12. Zaidi HA, Montoure AJ, Dickman CA. Surgical and clinical efficacy of sacroiliac joint fusion: a systematic review of the literature. J Neurosurg Spine 2015;23:59–66.
13. Ebraheim NA, Elgafy H, Semaan HB. Computed tomographic findings in patients with persistent sacroiliac pain after posterior iliac graft harvesting. Spine (Phila Pa 1976) 2000;25:2047–51.
14. Katz V, Schofferman J, Reynolds J. The sacroiliac joint: a potential cause of pain after lumbar fusion to the sacrum. J Spinal Disord Tech 2003;16:96–9.
15. Bernard TN Jr, Kirkaldy-Willis WH. Recognizing specific characteristics of nonspecific low back pain. Clin Orthop Relat Res 1987;(217):266–80.

16. Schwarzer AC, Aprill CN, Bogduk N. The sacroiliac joint in chronic low back pain. Spine (Phila Pa 1976) 1995;20:31–7.

17. Maigne JY, Aivaliklis A, Pfefer F. Results of sacroiliac joint double block and value of sacroiliac pain provocation tests in 54 patients with low back pain. Spine (Phila Pa 1976) 1996;21:1889–92.

18. Vleeming A, Schuenke MD, Masi AT, et al. The sacroiliac joint: an overview of its anatomy, function and potential clinical implications. J Anat 2012; 221:537–67.

19. Dreyfuss P, Dreyer SJ, Cole A, et al. Sacroiliac joint pain. J Am Acad Orthop Surg 2004;12:255–65.

20. Dreyfuss P, Michaelsen M, Pauza K, et al. The value of medical history and physical examination in diagnosing sacroiliac joint pain. Spine (Phila Pa 1976) 1996;21:2594–602.

21. Sturesson B, Selvik G, Uden A. Movements of the sacroiliac joints. A roentgen stereophotogrammetric analysis. Spine (Phila Pa 1976) 1989;14:162–5.

22. Roberts SL, Burnham RS, Ravichandiran K, et al. Cadaveric study of sacroiliac joint innervation: implications for diagnostic blocks and radiofrequency ablation. Reg Anesth Pain Med 2014;39: 456–64.

23. Forst SL, Wheeler MT, Fortin JD, et al. The sacroiliac joint: anatomy, physiology and clinical significance. Pain Physician 2006;9:61–7.

24. Grob KR, Neuhuber WL, Kissling RO. Innervation of the sacroiliac joint of the human. Z Rheumatol 1995; 54:117–22 [in German].

25. Chou LH, Slipman CW, Bhagia SM, et al. Inciting events initiating injection-proven sacroiliac joint syndrome. Pain Med 2004;5:26–32.

26. Slipman CW, Jackson HB, Lipetz JS, et al. Sacroiliac joint pain referral zones. Arch Phys Med Rehabil 2000;81:334–8.

27. Young S, Aprill C, Laslett M. Correlation of clinical examination characteristics with three sources of chronic low back pain. Spine J 2003;3:460–5.

28. Fortin JD, Falco FJ. The Fortin finger test: an indicator of sacroiliac pain. Am J Orthop (Belle Mead NJ) 1997;26:477–80.

29. Trescot AM. Cryoanalgesia in interventional pain management. Pain Physician 2003;6:345–60.

30. Cohen SP, Hurley RW, Buckenmaier CC 3rd, et al. Randomized placebo-controlled study evaluating lateral branch radiofrequency denervation for sacroiliac joint pain. Anesthesiology 2008; 109:279–88.

31. Patel N, Gross A, Brown L, et al. A randomized, placebo-controlled study to assess the efficacy of lateral branch neurotomy for chronic sacroiliac joint pain. Pain Med 2012;13:383–98.

32. Painter C. Excision of the Os innominatum: arthrodesis of the sacro-iliac synchrondosis. Boston Med Surg J 1908;159:205–8.

33. Smith-Petersen M. Arthrodesis of the sacroiliac joint. A new method of approach. J Orthop Surg 1921;3: 400–5.

34. Belanger TA, Dall BE. Sacroiliac arthrodesis using a posterior midline fascial splitting approach and pedicle screw instrumentation: a new technique. J Spinal Disord 2001;14:118–24.

35. Buchowski JM, Kebaish KM, Sinkov V, et al. Functional and radiographic outcome of sacroiliac arthrodesis for the disorders of the sacroiliac joint. Spine J 2005;5:520–8 [discussion: 529].

36. Giannikas KA, Khan AM, Karski MT, et al. Sacroiliac joint fusion for chronic pain: a simple technique avoiding the use of metalwork. Eur Spine J 2004; 13:253–6.

37. Polly DW, Cher DJ, Wine KD, et al. Randomized controlled trial of minimally invasive sacroiliac joint fusion using triangular titanium implants vs nonsurgical management for sacroiliac joint dysfunction: 12-month outcomes. Neurosurgery 2015;77:674–90 [discussion: 690–71].

38. Whang P, Cher D, Polly D, et al. Sacroiliac joint fusion using triangular titanium implants vs. nonsurgical management: six-month outcomes from a prospective randomized controlled trial. Int J Spine Surg 2015;9:6.

39. Rudolf L. Sacroiliac joint arthrodesis-MIS technique with titanium implants: report of the first 50 patients and outcomes. Open Orthop J 2012;6: 495–502.

40. Wise CL, Dall BE. Minimally invasive sacroiliac arthrodesis: outcomes of a new technique. J Spinal Disord Tech 2008;21:579–84.

41. Kibsgard TJ, Roise O, Stuge B. Pelvic joint fusion in patients with severe pelvic girdle pain—a prospective single-subject research design study. BMC Musculoskelet Disord 2014;15:85.

42. Beck CE, Jacobson S, Thomasson E. A retrospective outcomes study of 20 sacroiliac joint fusion patients. Cureus 2015;7:e260.

43. Polly DW, Swofford J, Whang PG, et al. Two-year outcomes from a randomized controlled trial of minimally invasive sacroiliac joint fusion vs. non-surgical management for sacroiliac joint dysfunction. Int J Spine Surg 2016;10:28.

44. Schutz U, Grob D. Poor outcome following bilateral sacroiliac joint fusion for degenerative sacroiliac joint syndrome. Acta Orthop Belg 2006;72: 296–308.

45. Lindsey DP, Perez-Orribo L, Rodriguez-Martinez N, et al. Evaluation of a minimally invasive procedure for sacroiliac joint fusion—an in vitro biomechanical analysis of initial and cycled properties. Med Devices (Auckl) 2014;7:131–7.

46. Leclercq TA. Posterior lumbar interbody fusion using the ray threaded fusion cage. J Clin Neurosci 1995; 2:129–31.

47. Ray CD. Threaded titanium cages for lumbar interbody fusions. Spine (Phila Pa 1976) 1997;22: 667–79 [discussion: 679–80].

48. Tullberg T, Brandt B, Rydberg J, et al. Fusion rate after posterior lumbar interbody fusion with carbon fiber implant: 1-year follow-up of 51 patients. Eur Spine J 1996;5:178–82.

49. Hitchon PW, Goel V, Rogge T, et al. Spinal stability with anterior or posterior ray threaded fusion cages. J Neurosurg 2000;93:102–8.

50. Kettler A, Wilke HJ, Dietl R, et al. Stabilizing effect of posterior lumbar interbody fusion cages before and after cyclic loading. J Neurosurg 2000;92:87–92.

51. McAfee PC, Cunningham BW, Lee GA, et al. Revision strategies for salvaging or improving failed cylindrical cages. Spine (Phila Pa 1976) 1999;24: 2147–53.

52. Onesti ST, Ashkenazi E. The ray threaded fusion cage for posterior lumbar interbody fusion. Neurosurgery 1998;42:200–4 [discussion: 204–5].

53. Tullberg T. Failure of a carbon fiber implant. A case report. Spine (Phila Pa 1976) 1998;23: 1804–6.

Is There Still a Role for Interspinous Spacers in the Management of Neurogenic Claudication?

CrossMark

Vijay M. Ravindra, MD, MSPH[a,b], Zoher Ghogawala, MD[b,c],*

KEYWORDS

- Neurogenic claudication • Interspinous spacer • Lumbar spinal stenosis

KEY POINTS

- Lumbar spinal stenosis with neurogenic claudication is a common condition and is the most common indication for spine surgery in patients over 65 years of age.
- Interspinous spacers provide a less invasive surgical option for patients suffering from mild-to-moderate lumbar spinal stenosis with intermittent neurogenic claudication.
- There is evidence of improvement in patient symptoms and outcomes at 1- and 2-year follow-up, but also a significant risk of needing reoperation (6%–85%).
- There may be a role for interspinous spacers for the management of neurogenic claudication, but strictly for patients without evidence of spondylolisthesis, severe osteoporosis, or adjacent-level neural foraminal stenosis and patients with mild-to-moderate lumbar spinal stenosis that is relieved with flexion maneuvers.
- Because the indications and contraindications are still unclear, future prospective study to identify the population that could most benefit from interspinous distraction is necessary.

INTRODUCTION

Lumbar spinal stenosis (LSS) and associated neurogenic claudication is a clinical syndrome of buttock or lower extremity pain with or without back pain that is a result of a decreased area for the neural and vascular structures present in the lumbar spine.[1] LSS can be congenital, but it is most commonly acquired in the setting of degenerative lumbar spine disease with associated facet hypertrophy and overgrown or hypertrophic ligamentum flavum seen with normal aging. It can also present after surgery or infection.[2,3] LSS with associated neurogenic claudication can cause significant chronic pain and disability, which leads to dramatic reduction in quality of life, mobility, and function.[2] In fact, LSS is one of the most common conditions referred to spinal subspecialists in the world and is the most common indication for spine surgery in patients over 65 years of age.[4]

Historically, surgical decompression has been a leading treatment for spinal stenosis and has offered significant improvement in patients' pain

Disclosures: None.
[a] Department of Neurosurgery, Clinical Neurosciences Center, University of Utah, 175 North Medical Drive East, Salt Lake City, UT 84132, USA; [b] Department of Neurosurgery, Alan and Jacqueline Stuart Spine Research Center, Lahey Hospital and Medical Center, 41 Mall Road, Burlington, MA 01805, USA; [c] Department of Neurosurgery, Tufts University School of Medicine, 145 Harrison Avenue, Boston, MA 02111, USA
* Corresponding author. Department of Neurosurgery, Alan and Jacqueline Stuart Spine Research Center, Lahey Hospital and Medical Center, 41 Mall Road, Burlington, MA 01805.
E-mail address: zoher.ghogawala@lahey.org

and function. In the 4-year analysis of the Spine Patient Outcomes Research Trial (SPORT) lumbar stenosis cohort, patients treated surgically had statistically improved Oswestry Disability Index (ODI) (9.4-point improvement), Short Form-36 (SF-36) bodily pain score (12.6-point improvement), and SF-36 physical function score (8.6-point improvement) compared with patients treated without surgery.[5] Similar results were found at 4 years in the Maine Lumbar Spine Study (MLSS), which demonstrated statistically greater satisfaction in surgically treated patients (63%) than in nonsurgically treated patients (42%).[6] The Finnish Lumbar Spinal Research Group reported improved ODI scores at 2 years among surgically treated patients in a randomized controlled trial comparing decompression and possible fusion versus nonoperative treatment.[7]

Although these results indicate good outcomes with surgical decompression, open surgery generally requires general anesthesia and can lead to instability,[8] and thus poses a significant risk to older patients. Minimally invasive surgical techniques and procedures have been developed to minimize morbidity while attempting to achieve similar results. Among these various techniques are interspinous process spacers, which offer an alternative to open surgical decompression for patients in whom nonsurgical treatment has failed.[9] This article reviews the current role of interspinous spacers in the treatment of neurogenic claudication and discusses the body of literature surrounding this treatment alternative.

INTERSPINOUS SPACER DEVELOPMENT

Interspinous process spacers were created as a less-invasive treatment option for spinal stenosis with neurogenic claudication for patients in whom conservative treatment measures have failed. Mechanical lumbar stenosis worsens with extension, so the spacer provides distraction of the spinous processes to limit extension, thus improving the symptoms associated with claudication.[9] Additional effects of distracting the neural foramen and unloading the intervertebral disc are also thought to improve central canal and foraminal stenosis.[10] The Wallis system (Abbott Spine, Austin, Texas) was the first interspinous process spacer developed, in 1986; it was primarily used for patients with recurrent disc herniation.[11,12] In 2005, the X-Stop Interspinous Process Decompression System (St. Francis Medical Technologies, Concord, California) received U.S. Food and Drug Administration (FDA) approval for treatment of neurogenic claudication secondary to LSS (**Fig. 1**).[1] No additional interspinous process

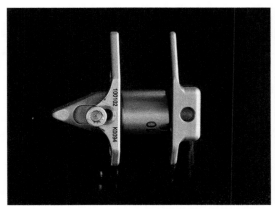

Fig. 1. Photograph of the X-stop device, the original interspinous spacer device that received FDA approval for the treatment of LSS with neurogenic claudication in 2005. (*From* Bowers C, Amini A, Dailey AT, et al. Dynamic interspinous process stabilization: review of complications associated with the X-Stop device. Neurosurg Focus 2010;28(6):E8; with permission.)

spacers have been approved by the FDA, although there are other commercially available devices used for similar indications (**Table 1**).

Neurophysiologic study of interspinous distraction also supports the use of distraction for LSS. Schizas and colleagues[17] found that distraction of 8 mm was sufficient to replicate electrophysiological improvements during full decompression, although not in multilevel LSS. Thus, interspinous distraction does have a measurable neurophysiological effect, likely lending to its efficacy and improvement in symptoms across multiple studies.

SURGICAL VERSUS NONSURGICAL MANAGEMENT OF LUMBAR SPINAL STENOSIS

LSS has a significant impact on mobility, functioning, and quality of life, and its prevalence will continue to rise as the population ages.[18] Currently, nonsurgical management of LSS with neurogenic intermittent claudication includes judicious use of anti-inflammatory medications, physical therapy programs, and epidural steroid injections.[19] There is low-quality evidence that shows that surgical decompression and conservative treatment have similar results in regards to disability (ODI) at 3, 6, and 12 months.[7,20,21] However, the high- quality SPORT trial reported better outcomes at 2 and 4 years for surgical decompression.[20]

Nonsurgical management of LSS has a low complication rate, whereas 10% to 24% of

Table 1
List of interspinous process spacers, indications, and FDA approval status

Device (Manufacturer)	Indication	FDA Approved
Wallis (Abbott Spine, Austin, Texas)[11,12]	Degenerative disk disease, lateral recess, and central spinal stenosis	No
X-Stop (St. Francis Medical Technologies, Concord, California)[13]	Lumbar spinal stenosis with neurogenic claudication	Yes
DIAM (Sofamor Danek, Memphis, Tennesee)[14]	Lumbar spinal stenosis	No
Coflex (Paradigm Spine, New York, New York)[15,16]	Lumbar spinal stenosis	Yes
Superion (Vertiflex Inc., San Clemente, California)[9]	Lumbar spinal stenosis with neurogenic claudication	No

Data from Refs.[9,11–16]

patients who have undergone surgical decompression experience complications.[7,20,21] A glaring shortcoming of studies examining the efficacy of conservative management is the lack of uniformity among conservative treatment methods. In a Cochrane review, Zaina and colleagues[18] noted the discrepancy in modalities applied for conservative treatment and recommended that future studies should isolate specific approaches with clearly defined treatment plans. Involvement of pain management specialists, physiatrists, and primary care physicians in these studies could help delineate specific treatment plans that may be beneficial.

Surgical management options include decompression, decompression with fusion, and interspinous process distraction, a minimally invasive surgical option. Although decompression without fusion may be considered the gold standard in the treatment of LSS, there are patients who are not satisfied with their outcomes after surgery.[5,22–24] This has led some surgeons to increase their use of spinal fusion or to explore minimally invasive treatment options. Recent Level I evidence by Ghogawala and colleagues[25] comparing treatment options demonstrated that patients with Grade I spondylolisthesis with LSS who underwent decompression and fusion had a greater increase in SF-36 physical-component summary scores at 2 years after surgery than the decompression-alone group ($P = .046$), a difference that remained at 3 and 4 years ($P = .02$). There was a nonsignificant difference in reduction in disability (ODI) between the 2 groups at 4 years ($P = .05$). Although blood loss and hospital stay were longer for the fusion cohort, the cumulative rate of reoperation was lower (14% vs 34%, $P = .05$).[25] Another recent report demonstrated that the use of fusion in patients with lumbar spinal stenosis with or without degenerative

spondylolisthesis did not result in better clinical outcomes at 2 and 5 years.[26] Furthermore, there is evidence that demonstrates that the addition of fusion to decompression can significantly increase complication rates.[4] Decompressive techniques are also evolving; Thome and colleagues[27] additionally showed the outcome of bilateral laminotomy is more beneficial than conventional laminectomy.

There is an obvious advantage to avoiding an open operation, including shorter hospitalization and better healing from muscle dissection. In addition to devices placed with a smaller incision, the percutaneous delivery of a device (Aperius PercLID, Medrontic Kyphon, Pfaeffikon, Switzerland)[28] has also been described; its use resulted in improvements in visual analog scale (VAS) and Zurich Claudication Questionnaire scores for patients with low back pain and leg pain and neurogenic claudication.

CONFLICTING EVIDENCE FOR INTERSPINOUS SPACER USE

Initial reports about the success of X-Stop device in 2005 increased its popularity. Zucherman and colleagues[13] reported the results of a multicenter, prospective, randomized trial of interspinous process device implantation. The trial included 191 patients diagnosed with painful neurogenic claudication; patients treated with the X-Stop device (intervention group) had significantly greater pain control than those treated with epidural steroid injections (control group) at the 1- and 2-year time points. There was a 6% revision rate in patients who received X-Stop devices. Although these data show superiority for the interspinous process device, the results and comparison should be interpreted carefully, especially since the control group was treated with epidural steroid injections, which is not the therapy of choice for LSS with neurogenic claudication. This was followed by the report from Siddiqi and colleagues,[29] who reported a revision rate of under 10%. At 1-year follow-up, 54% of patients reported clinically significant improvement in their symptoms; 33% had improvement in their physical function, and 71% were satisfied with the procedure, although 29% of patients required a caudal epidural for recurrence of the symptoms of neurogenic claudication.[29]

Stromqvist and colleagues[30] compared the X-Stop device with decompressive surgery for lumbar neurogenic intermittent claudication in a randomized controlled trial with 2 years of clinical follow-up and determined that both procedures were appropriate for the treatment of neurogenic claudication. The primary (Zurich Claudication Questionnaire) and secondary (VAS, SF-36, complications, and reoperations) outcome measures were similar at 6, 12, and 24 months. Further surgery was necessary in 3 patients in the surgical decompression group (6%) and 13 patents (26%) in the X-Stop group ($P = .04$) suggesting limited durability of the X-Stop device.

Tuschel and colleagues[31] found an alarmingly high revision rate of 30.4% in a series of 46 patients treated with the X-Stop interspinous process distraction device. They associated lack of improvement at 6-week follow-up with subsequent revision surgery, which usually took place 12 months after the initial intervention. It is noteworthy that the clinical outcome parameters improved significantly for the patients who did not require reoperation, with a Kaplan-Meier survivorship analysis predicting implant survival probability of 0.68 at 2 years postoperatively.[31] The high revision rate in this series may have been secondary to longer follow-up, and the authors posited that outcomes, specifically revision rates, may be less favorable than initially reported.

Along with skepticism about outcomes based on early trial results came biomechanical concerns about the use of interspinous spacer devices. Initially, there was some concern about the potential for the devices to push the spine into a kyphotic position, but Schulete and colleagues[19] demonstrated that overall sagittal balance was not affected after the use of interspinous spacers in a cohort of 20 patients, and, in fact, interspinous spacers may improve overall spinal alignment. More recently, Bae and colleagues[32] reported the 3-year results of a prospective, randomized investigational trial comparing Coflex interlaminar stabilization versus instrumented fusion in patients with lumbar stenosis. In this study, there were comparable improvements in patient-reported outcomes in both groups, although a higher percentage of patients in the Coflex group reported a clinically significant improvement (≥ 15) in ODI ($P = .008$). Radiographic measurements demonstrated maintenance of adjacent-level range of motion in patients who had Coflex interlaminar stabilization, although range of motion at the level superior to fusion was significantly increased ($P = .005$). The conclusions of this most recent study suggest that Coflex Interlaminar Stabilization for stenosis is effective and durable at improving overall composite clinical success without altering normal spinal kinematic motion at the index level of decompression or adjacent levels.[32]

INDICATIONS FOR INTERSPINOUS SPACER USE

Although there are several Level I studies proving that interspinous process spacer devices are useful, less-invasive surgical options for the treatment of lumbar spinal stenosis, there is an overall lack of consensus regarding clear indications, and, more importantly, contraindications for the procedure. Nevertheless, Siewe and colleagues[33] have recently compiled the results of a questionnaire sent to experienced spine surgeons that suggests conditions for which interspinous process spacer devices may (or may not) be indicated (**Box 1**).

Box 1
Updated list of general indications and contraindications for the use of interspinous process spacer devices

Indications

- Age greater than 50 years
- Pain or symptoms relieved with flexion maneuvers
- Foraminal stenosis at the affected level without significant adjacent-level foraminal stenosis
- Mild or moderate LSS with neurogenic claudication
- Previously mentioned characteristics, not able to tolerate general anesthesia

Contraindications

- Disease spanning greater than 2 segments
- Infection
- Fracture
- Isthmic spondylolisthesis
- Degenerative spondylolisthesis
- Lumbar spine scoliosis
- Osteoporosis or severe osteopenia

SURGICAL TECHNIQUE/PROCEDURE

The technique for placement of interspinous spacer devices may vary by device manufacturer, but the general principles are the same. The procedure is undertaken in the operating room, where patients are placed in the lateral decubitus or prone position and asked to flex their spine (**Fig. 2**). The level and interspinous space to be targeted are then localized with intraoperative fluoroscopy. Most patients undergo this procedure with local anesthetic with intravenous sedation as an adjunct; general anesthesia is not typically required.

The incision is located in the midsagittal location over the spinous process of the targeted level. Incision length can vary, but on average it is 4 cm in length. The paraspinal tissue and musculature are elevated to the level of the laminar arch and facet joints. In severe cases of degenerative disease and arthritis, hypertrophied facet joints that impede access to the anterior interspinous space are trimmed to enable anterior placement of the implant.[34] A dilator is then inserted to the anterior margin of the interspinous space to pierce the interspinous ligament. A sizer is used to determine the size of the implant to be used. The interspinous spacer device is then secured to the insertion device and driven into the interspinous space. The goal is to place the device as close to the posterior aspect of the lamina as possible. The incision is then closed. Theoretically, patients who tolerate the procedure well, with limited comorbidities, are able to go home the same day (**Fig. 3**).[34]

SURGICAL COMPLICATIONS AND MANAGEMENT

Although interspinous process spacers provide an attractive alternative to surgical decompression, there are complications associated with their use. The most commonly reported complications are device dislocation, spinous process fractures, spinous process erosion,[35] infection, hematoma, and neurologic symptoms, such as foot drop (**Table 2**).[36]

The early randomized prospective study of the X-Stop device by Zucherman and colleagues[13] had a 4% complication rate and a reoperation rate of 6% in 100 patients, but subsequent studies have reported more complications and failures secondary to these devices (**Table 3**). As a result, there has been an appeal for additional reports of negative results from the use of X-Stop device.[37] Complication rates as high as 38%[10] have been

reported from the use of interspinous process spacers. Reoperation rates ranging from 6% to 85% have been reported specifically for the X-Stop device.[10,13]

As with any medical device, interspinous spacers have been modified in their use, indications, and contraindications over the years. Verhoof and colleagues[38] described the use of the X-Stop device for patients with Grade I spondylolisthesis and reported a 58% failure/reoperation rate. These findings led to the conclusion that this device should not be used in spondylolisthesis, which is now listed as a strict contraindication for the device.

Spinous process fractures can occur with immediate placement of the device or in a delayed manner. Delayed spinous process fractures with the device have been described in the setting of the sandwich phenomenon, which refers to a fracture of the middle spinous process in adjacent double-level X-Stop placement.[39] The reason for acute or delayed fracture is not specifically known, but it likely relates to poor bone quality and overdistraction or overdilation. Thus, preoperative measurement of bone density and surgical planning are necessary to minimize the risks. Overdistraction can also lead to radiculopathy, typically 1 level above the treated level. Wiseman and colleagues[40] demonstrated that interspinous spacers unload the facet joints at the affected levels while causing an increase in the adjacent peak pressure by nearly 20%. The increased pressure on the adjacent facet, adjacent neural foraminal stenosis, and a large implant that is overdistracted may be enough to exacerbate adjacent-level radiculopathy.[10]

In addition to a steep learning curve with the use of interspinous spacer devices, patient selection remains variable through a large number of studies. As mentioned previously, it has been suggested that use of interspinous spacer devices in patients with Grade I spondylolisthesis should be avoided. Additionally, the use of this technology may be limited to those with mild-to-moderate lumbar canal stenosis, thus excluding those with severe lumbar spinal stenosis.[41] An additional factor may lie in the selection of patients who have clear demonstration of positional-dependent claudication relieved by flexion.[42]

FUTURE DIRECTIONS AND CONSENSUS STATEMENT

Despite multiple reports of significant complications occurring at alarming rates, there are a

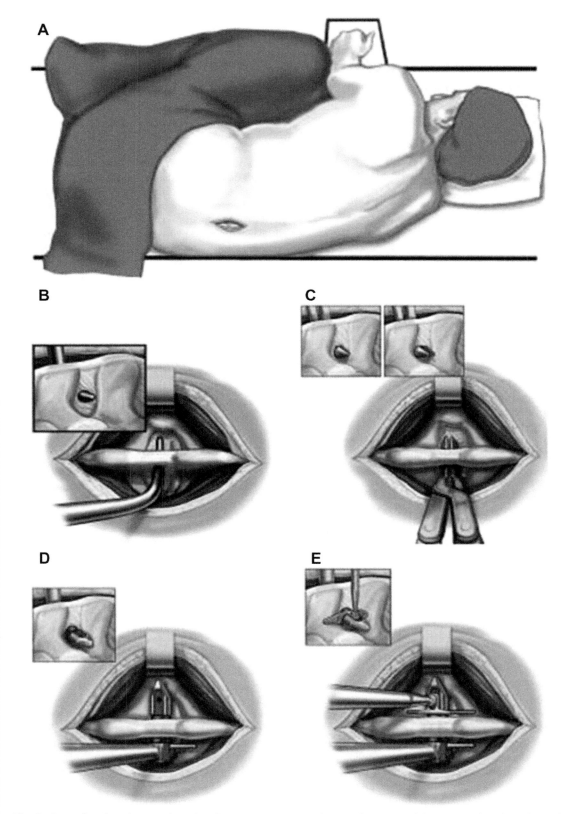

Fig. 2. Example of patient undergoing interspinous spacer device placement. (*A*) Patient placed in the right lateral decubitus position with an incision at the stenotic level. (*B*) Curved dilator placed in the anterior margin of the interspinous space. (*C*) Sizing distractor inserted to determine implant size. (*D*) Device inserted into the interspinous space. (*E*) Adjustable components fastened to the implant to prevent dislodging. (*From* Zucherman JF, Hsu KY, Hartjen CA, et al. A prospective randomized multi-center study for the treatment of lumbar spinal stenosis with the X STOP interspinous implant: 1-year results. Eur Spine J 2004;13(1):23; with permission.)

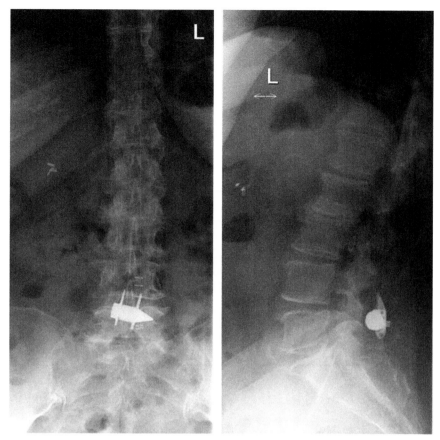

Fig. 3. Postoperative anterior/posterior (*left*) and lateral (*right*) radiographs after interspinous process spacer placement.

number of randomized prospective, case series, biomechanical, and physiologic studies that demonstrate the potential positive effects of the use of interspinous spacers. Careful patient selection and counseling are needed to ascertain which patients would benefit most from this intervention. It is likely there is still a role for interspinous spacers for the management of neurogenic claudication from lumbar spinal stenosis, but strictly for patients without evidence of spondylolisthesis, severe osteoporosis, or adjacent-level neural foraminal stenosis and for patients with mild-to-moderate lumbar spinal stenosis that is relieved with flexion maneuvers. Future prospective study targeting this specific population could be useful in clarifying the potential durable effect of interspinous distraction.

Table 2
Complications associated with the interspinous process devices

Complication	Timing	Consequence
Device dislocation	Immediate or delayed	Pain
Spinous process fractures	Immediate or delayed	Pain
Spinous process erosion	Delayed	Pain
Infection	Delayed	Pain, systemic illness
Hematoma	Immediate	Pain, neurologic deficit
Nerve root compression from overdistration	Immediate or delayed	Pain, neurologic deficit

Table 3
Large series of interspinous process spacer use and associated complications

Study	Number of Patients	Follow-up (mo)	Number (%) of Patients with Complications	Number (%) of Patients Requiring Additional Surgery	Number or % of Patients Achieving Good Outcome
Zucherman et al,[13] 2005	100	24	4 (4%)	6 (6%)	73.1%
Siddiqui et al,[29] 2007	24	12	2 (5%) spinous process fractures	2 (8%)	Improvement in pain (54%); improvement in physical function (33%)
Verhoof et al,[38] 2008	12	30	0	7 (58%)	5 (42%)
Brussee et al,[43] 2008	65	12	0	6 (9%)	20 (31%)
Barbagallo et al,[44] 2009	69	23	4 (6%) spinous process fractures; 4 (6%) device dislocations	5 (7%)	NA
Bowers et al,[10] 2010	13	46	3 (23%) spinous process fractures; 2 (15%) radiculopathy	11 (85%)	2 (15%)
Tuschel et al,[31] 2013	46	40	0	14 (30.4%)	25 (84%)

Abbreviation: N/A, not available.
  Data from Refs.[10,13,29,31,38,43,44]

SUMMARY

Interspinous spacer devices offer a less invasive surgical option for patients experiencing mild-to-moderate lumbar spinal stenosis with intermittent neurogenic claudication, and some evidence supports improvement in patient symptoms and outcome in some situations. This procedure may be advantageous in those with good bone quality, absence of adjacent-level foraminal stenosis, and true positional symptoms that are relieved with flexion. The current literature on the topic demonstrates that symptom relief may be significant, but there are significant concerns regarding durability, with significant numbers of patients undergoing reoperation (6%–85%). Careful patient selection and preoperative counseling are necessary prior to recommending interspinous spacer device implantation.

REFERENCES

1. Watters WC 3rd, Baisden J, Gilbert TJ, et al. Degenerative lumbar spinal stenosis: an evidence-based clinical guideline for the diagnosis and treatment of degenerative lumbar spinal stenosis. Spine J 2008; 8(2):305–10.

2. Chad DA. Lumbar spinal stenosis. Neurol Clin 2007; 25(2):407–18.

3. Ciricillo SF, Weinstein PR. Lumbar spinal stenosis. West J Med 1993;158(2):171–7.

4. Deyo RA, Mirza SK, Martin BI, et al. Trends, major medical complications, and charges associated with surgery for lumbar spinal stenosis in older adults. JAMA 2010;303(13):1259–65.

5. Weinstein JN, Tosteson TD, Lurie JD, et al. Surgical versus nonoperative treatment for lumbar spinal stenosis four-year results of the Spine Patient Outcomes Research Trial. Spine (Phila Pa 1976) 2010; 35(14):1329–38.

6. Atlas SJ, Keller RB, Wu YA, et al. Long-term outcomes of surgical and nonsurgical management of lumbar spinal stenosis: 8 to 10 year results from the Maine lumbar spine study. Spine (Phila Pa 1976) 2005;30(8):936–43.

7. Malmivaara A, Slatis P, Heliovaara M, et al. Surgical or nonoperative treatment for lumbar spinal stenosis? A randomized controlled trial. Spine (Phila Pa 1976) 2007;32(1):1–8.

8. Trouillier H, Birkenmaier C, Kluzik J, et al. Operative treatment for degenerative lumbar spinal canal stenosis. Acta Orthop Belg 2004;70(4):337–43.

9. Patel VV, Whang PG, Haley TR, et al. Superion interspinous process spacer for intermittent neurogenic

claudication secondary to moderate lumbar spinal stenosis: two-year results from a randomized controlled FDA-IDE pivotal trial. Spine (Phila Pa 1976) 2015;40(5):275–82.

10. Bowers C, Amini A, Dailey AT, et al. Dynamic interspinous process stabilization: review of complications associated with the X-Stop device. Neurosurg Focus 2010;28(6):E8.

11. Senegas J. Mechanical supplementation by nonrigid fixation in degenerative intervertebral lumbar segments: the Wallis system. Eur Spine J 2002; 11(Suppl 2):S164–9.

12. Boeree N. Dynamic stabilization of the degenerative lumbar motion segment: the Wallis system. Spine J 2005;54(4):S89–90.

13. Zucherman JF, Hsu KY, Hartjen CA, et al. A multicenter, prospective, randomized trial evaluating the X STOP interspinous process decompression system for the treatment of neurogenic intermittent claudication: two-year follow-up results. Spine (Phila Pa 1976) 2005;30(12):1351–8.

14. Guizzardi G, Petriini P, Fabrizi A, et al. The use of DIAM (interspinous stress-breaker device) in the DDD: Italian multicenter clinical experience. Paper presented at 5th Annual Meeting: Spinal Arthoplasty Society. New York, NY, May 4–7, 2005.

15. Eif M, Schenke H. The Interspinous-U: Indications, experience, and results. Paper presented at 5th Annual Meeting: Spinal Arthroplasty Society. New York, NY, May 4–7, 2005.

16. Cho K-S. Clinical outcome of the Interspinous-U (posterior distraction device) in the elderly lumbar spine. Paper presented at 5th Annual Meeting: Spinal Arthroplasty Society, New York, NY, May 4–7, 2005.

17. Schizas C, Pralong E, Tzioupis C, et al. Interspinous distraction in lumbar spinal stenosis: a neurophysiological perspective. Spine (Phila Pa 1976) 2013; 38(24):2113–7.

18. Zaina F, Tomkins-Lane C, Carragee E, et al. Surgical versus nonsurgical treatment for lumbar spinal stenosis. Spine (Phila Pa 1976) 2016;41(14):E857–68.

19. Schulte LM, O'Brien JR, Matteini LE, et al. Change in sagittal balance with placement of an interspinous spacer. Spine (Phila Pa 1976) 2011;36(20):E1302–5.

20. Weinstein JN, Tosteson TD, Lurie JD, et al. Surgical versus nonsurgical therapy for lumbar spinal stenosis. N Engl J Med 2008;358(8):794–810.

21. Amundsen T, Weber H, Nordal HJ, et al. Lumbar spinal stenosis: conservative or surgical management?: A prospective 10-year study. Spine (Phila Pa 1976) 2000;25(11):1424–35 [discussion: 1435–6].

22. Weinstein JN, Lurie JD, Tosteson TD, et al. Surgical compared with nonoperative treatment for lumbar degenerative spondylolisthesis. four-year results in the Spine Patient Outcomes Research Trial (SPORT) randomized and observational cohorts. J Bone Joint Surg Am 2009;91(6):1295–304.

23. Turner JA, Ersek M, Herron L, et al. Surgery for lumbar spinal stenosis. Attempted meta-analysis of the literature. Spine (Phila Pa 1976) 1992;17(1):1–8.

24. Jonsson B, Annertz M, Sjoberg C, et al. A prospective and consecutive study of surgically treated lumbar spinal stenosis. Part II: five-year follow-up by an independent observer. Spine (Phila Pa 1976) 1997;22(24):2938–44.

25. Ghogawala Z, Dziura J, Butler WE, et al. Laminectomy plus fusion versus laminectomy alone for lumbar spondylolisthesis. N Engl J Med 2016;374(15): 1424–34.

26. Forsth P, Olafsson G, Carlsson T, et al. A randomized, controlled trial of fusion surgery for lumbar spinal stenosis. N Engl J Med 2016; 374(15):1413–23.

27. Thome C, Zevgaridis D, Leheta O, et al. Outcome after less-invasive decompression of lumbar spinal stenosis: a randomized comparison of unilateral laminotomy, bilateral laminotomy, and laminectomy. J Neurosurg Spine 2005;3(2):129–41.

28. Nardi P, Cabezas D, Rea G, et al. Aperius PercLID stand alone interspinous system for the treatment of degenerative lumbar stenosis: experience on 152 cases. J Spinal Disord Tech 2010; 23(3):203–7.

29. Siddiqui M, Smith FW, Wardlaw D. One-year results of X Stop interspinous implant for the treatment of lumbar spinal stenosis. Spine (Phila Pa 1976) 2007;32(12):1345–8.

30. Stromqvist BH, Berg S, Gerdhem P, et al. X-stop versus decompressive surgery for lumbar neurogenic intermittent claudication: randomized controlled trial with 2-year follow-up. Spine (Phila Pa 1976) 2013;38(17): 1436–42.

31. Tuschel A, Chavanne A, Eder C, et al. Implant survival analysis and failure modes of the X-Stop interspinous distraction device. Spine (Phila Pa 1976) 2013;38(21):1826–31.

32. Bae HW, Davis RJ, Lauryssen C, et al. Three-year follow-up of the prospective, randomized, controlled trial of coflex interlaminar stabilization vs instrumented fusion in patients with lumbar stenosis. Neurosurgery 2016;79(2):169–81.

33. Siewe J, Selbeck M, Koy T, et al. Indications and contraindications: interspinous process decompression devices in lumbar spine surgery. J Neurol Surg A Cent Eur Neurosurg 2015;76(1):1–7.

34. Zucherman JF, Hsu KY, Hartjen CA, et al. A prospective randomized multi-center study for the treatment of lumbar spinal stenosis with the X STOP interspinous implant: 1-year results. Eur Spine J 2004;13(1):22–31.

35. Miller JD, Miller MC, Lucas MG. Erosion of the spinous process: a potential cause of interspinous process spacer failure. J Neurosurg Spine 2010; 12(2):210–3.

36. Epstein NE. X-Stop: foot drop. Spine J 2009;9(5): e6–9.

37. Epstein NE. How often is minimally invasive minimally effective: what are the complication rates for minimally invasive surgery? Surg Neurol 2008; 70(4):386–8 [discussion: 389].

38. Verhoof OJ, Bron JL, Wapstra FH, et al. High failure rate of the interspinous distraction device (X-Stop) for the treatment of lumbar spinal stenosis caused by degenerative spondylolisthesis. Eur Spine J 2008;17(2):188–92.

39. Barbagallo GM, Corbino LA, Olindo G, et al. The "sandwich phenomenon": a rare complication in adjacent, double-level X-stop surgery: report of three cases and review of the literature. Spine (Phila Pa 1976) 2010;35(3):E96–100.

40. Wiseman CM, Lindsey DP, Fredrick AD, et al. The effect of an interspinous process implant on facet loading during extension. Spine (Phila Pa 1976) 2005;30(8):903–7.

41. Eichholz KM, Fessler RG. Is the X STOP interspinous implant a safe and effective treatment for neurogenic intermittent claudication? Nat Clin Pract Neurol 2006;2(1):22–3.

42. Kuchta J, Sobottke R, Eysel P, et al. Two-year results of interspinous spacer (X-Stop) implantation in 175 patients with neurologic intermittent claudication due to lumbar spinal stenosis. Eur Spine J 2009; 18(6):823–9.

43. Brussee P, Hauth J, Donk RD, et al. Self-rated evaluation of outcome of the implantation of interspinous process distraction (X-Stop) for neurogenic claudication. Eur Spine J 2008;17(2):200–3.

44. Barbagallo GM, Corbino LA, Olindo G, et al. Analysis of complications in patients treated with the X-Stop Interspinous Process Decompression System: proposal for a novel anatomic scoring system for patient selection and review of the literature. Neurosurgery 2009;65:111–20.

Bone Morphogenic Protein Use in Spinal Surgery

John F. Burke, MD, PhD, Sanjay S. Dhall, MD*

KEYWORDS

- Bone morphogenic protein • Spinal surgery • Fusion • Ethical standards

KEY POINTS

- Bone morphogenic protein (BMP) provides excellent enhancement of fusion in many spinal surgeries.
- BMP should be a cautionary tale about the use of industry-sponsored research, perceived conflicts of interest, and holding the field of spinal surgery to the highest academic scrutiny and ethical standards.
- In the case of BMP, not having a transparent base of literature as it was approved led to delays in allowing this superior technology to help patients.

INTRODUCTION

Spinal surgery has been increasingly used over the last several decades in order to correct structural compression of neural elements. The goal of spinal surgery is 2-fold: to decompress neural elements and to fuse the bony elements surrounding the spine to prevent future instability.

In particular, there are 2 methods used to promote bony fusion across adjacent vertebral elements. The first method is referred to as "instrumentation-induced fusion (IIF)." In this method, hardware is affixed to the bony elements of the spine to immobilize them relative to each other. Fusion then results over several months as bone formation occurs across these immobilized bony elements.

Another method involves the placement of material adjacent to the vertebrae to enhance bone growth, which is referred to as "material-induced fusion (MIF)." Importantly, MIF is completely independent of IIF, and each of these methods can be performed separately from or simultaneously with the other. As an example, "on-lay fusion" techniques represent MIF performed separately from IIF. However, placing pedicle screws and rods in conjunction with iliac bone autograft for lumbar spinal fusion represents the simultaneous use of MIF and IIF techniques. Importantly, the gold standard of MIF is the use of iliac bone autograft to enhance bony fusion. However, iliac bone autograft has been associated with a relatively high morbidity and leads to often unacceptable levels of postoperative pain that can impede recovery and prolong hospital length of stay.

The use of bone morphogenic protein (BMP) has thus been proposed to replace iliac bone autograft to enhance bony fusion. It is important to view the use of BMP within the broad goals of spine surgery: it is one method to enhance arthrodesis. In that context, it is not important to determine if BMP enhances bone growth, but instead it is

Disclosure of Funding: Dr S.S. Dhall, MD receives honoraria from Depuy Spine and Globus Medical.
Conflicts of Interest: The authors declare no competing conflicts of interest.
Department of Neurological Surgery, University of California, San Francisco, 505 Parnassus Avenue, Room M779, San Francisco, CA 94143-0112, USA
* Corresponding author.
E-mail address: sanjaydhall@gmail.com

important to determine if BMP promotes arthrodesis at a higher rate than other MIF and IIF approaches within an acceptable safety profile.

BMP itself is a salient topic in spine surgery, primarily because it has gained widespread use. Indeed, many spine surgeons across both neurosurgery as well as orthopedic surgery use BMP as a method of MIF despite the fact that BMP has not gained general US Food and Drug Administration (FDA) approval for this purpose. As a result, most surgeons have adopted the practice of adding the off-label use of BMP to the consenting process for surgery. With such widespread adoption by the spine community without the express sanctioning by the FDA, it remains the responsibility of those in the field of spinal surgery to continuously weigh the risks and benefits of BMP. Such heightened scrutiny is especially needed because BMP has an unclear safety profile, and it is argued to be a nontrivial cause of various numbers of postoperative complications and adverse events.

In this review, the authors first review the development of BMP. Then, they cover the controversy surrounding the role of BMP in the development of bony cancers. Finally, the authors summarize the current state of affairs regarding the use of BMP in spinal surgery.

DEVELOPMENT OF BONE MORPHOGENIC PROTEIN

BMP, or recombinant human bone morphogenic protein-2, was initially discovered in the 1960s by Marshall Urist.[1] It was introduced as a commercial product in 2002 for the purpose of increasing the rate of bony fusion after spinal surgery. Commercially, BMP is used through BMP-impregnated collagen sponges, creating an implantable substance that is placed in the vicinity of bone in order to induce bony fusion. Strong preclinical data supporting the use of BMP to enhance growth of existing bone appeared in the literature in the 1990s.[2] The first human trials testing the correct dosing and the safety profile of BMP occurred in the late 1990s, 2000,[2] and 2002.[3] These data were quickly followed by industry-supported research that endorsed the use of BMP in spinal surgery, and all reported an excellent safety profile. Specifically, Boden and colleagues[4] used BMP in anterior lumbar interbody fusions (ALIFs) in 11 patients and found that BMP enhanced the rate of bony fusion. Boden and colleagues[3] also used BMP in posterior spinal fusions and found a similar result. Burkus and colleagues[5,6] produced several articles using BMP in ALIFs, again finding that BMP led increased rate of fusion. Similarly, many other

articles, all reporting on trials that were funded from industry, found similar positive results for BMP and, in general, reported no adverse affects related to BMP.[7–9] Based on these results, a meta-analysis of the use of BMP reported that industry-led research tested the use of BMP on 780 patients and reported a 0% rate of adverse events, suggesting that BMP has at most a 0.5% adverse event rate within 99% confidence intervals.[10]

Based on a subset of these data, BMP was approved by the FDA for use in spinal surgery. However, the use of BMP in spine surgery was approved only for one-level ALIFs with very particular types of cages that were used in the industry-sponsored clinical data. Specifically, the cages had to be tapered and threaded and included a lordotic curvature. Of note, most of the clinical data from the industry trials tested the use of BMP in ALIFs, which explains the reasoning of the FDA to approve BMP for just that purpose. Later on in 2004, the FDA approved the use of BMP in revision surgeries for posterior lateral interbody fusions as well.

After this approval, there were naturally many studies that were geared toward showing that BMP could be safely used in indications other than one-level ALIFs. Thus, this led to the state of affairs from 2010 to the present day in which BMP was frequently used off label for posterior and transforaminal lumbar interbody fusions as well as in thoracic and cervical procedures such as anterior cervical discectomy and fusions (ACDFs).

CONTROVERSY SURROUNDING BONE MORPHOGENIC PROTEIN USE

Based on skepticism of industry-led clinical trials, the incredibly low adverse event rate associated with BMP, the speed with which BMP achieved FDA approval, and the widespread off-label use of BMP in spine surgery, studies began to reexamine the safety profile of BMP.

Concerns first started to mount when anecdotal data supported the idea that BMP use in ACDF led to an increased inflammatory response of cervical prevertebral tissue. This increase in prevertebral soft tissue swelling led to an increased rate of dyspnea and dysphagia in the postoperative period. In severe cases, the increased prevertebral soft tissue swelling led to emergent intubation in order to prevent respiratory collapse.

As a result, these reports and other concerns led to the FDA issuing a public health notification on the use of BMP in June 2008. In that public health notification, the FDA cited that the use of BMP caused an immune-type reaction that led to the swelling of the airway and laryngeal edema that, in certain cases, needed to be treated with intubation and tracheotomy. In short order, this led to an investigation of Medtronic, the principal producer of BMP, by the Justice Department.

As concerns began to mount, more articles regarding the use of BMP were published. These articles suggested that BMP caused a wide range of adverse events, including migration of implants, increase in local inflammation, increase in infection risk, increase in ectopic bone formation, as well as the most concerning complication of induction bony carcinogenesis of the bone. Aside from these outright safety concerns, there have been more protocol-driven concerns about the appropriate dosing for a given spinal procedure. Given the relatively high rate of BMP used in an off-label fashion, there is great concern regarding the appropriate dose for different spinal surgeries and how to titrate the correct dose to optimize the risk benefit profile of BMP.

After several other allegations about the veracity of clinical trials using BMP in human studies, there was a retraction of a prominent article supporting the use of BMP, after the methods were called into question and the lead surgeon on the study was found to have inappropriate industry-related financial ties.[12,13]

Based on the rising controversy surrounding the use of BMP, the *Spine Journal* published a re-review of the original industry-sponsored trials as well as all of the human studies examining the use of BMP in 2011.[10] These investigators found that, of the original 13 industry-sponsored trials of BMP, there were methodological biases against the control group when examining the use of BMP in posterior and posterior-lateral interbody fusions. The study also found that these articles inflated the morbidity associated with the gold standard for fusions—iliac bone autograft. Indeed, some of the original industry-led studies found that iliac bone autograft had a morbidity ranging from 40% to 60%. Finally, the study examined previously unpublished data and found that the actual rate of adverse affects associated with the use of BMP ranged from 10% to 50%. In addition, the use of BMP in ACDF procedures indeed led to increased rate of adverse events. The study found that the adverse events associated with BMP included a higher rate of infection, implant displacement, and subsidence, as well as radiculitis and worse overall outcomes, in addition to many other adverse events.[10]

THE CURRENT USE OF BONE MORPHOGENIC PROTEIN

BMP has clearly inspired a lively debate about usage in spinal surgery. At the heart of the debate lies the history that led to the development of BMP. Specifically, the original articles that supported the use of BMP had ties to industry and suffered perceived conflicts of interest regarding the approval of BMP. In this regard, BMP approval and off-label use represent a teaching point that we, as spine surgeons, can use to promote the highest ethical standards in the field of spinal surgery. BMP use offers an effective method for promoting bony fusion after spine surgery; however, the initial data that introduced BMP were not free of conflict of interest, and, as a result, it is the responsibility of the spine surgery community to hold the use of BMP to the absolute most critical and rigorous scientific and ethical standards.

A recent study was designed to critically appraise the use of BMP in spine surgery. Hofstetter and colleagues[11] (2016) aggregated data from the use of BMP across a wide range of spinal surgical procedures. The investigators found that the use of BMP at the lowest dose (0.2–0.6 mg per level) enhanced fusion at a rate similar to higher doses and was not associated with an increased adverse event rate at higher doses. In addition, the use of such low-dose BMP in ACDF resulted in a significantly higher rate of fusion than control groups (98% vs 85%) for multilevel ACDFs; however, there was no difference in fusion rate for single-level ACDFs. Thus, it seems reasonable to use BMP in multilevel ACDFs at the lowest possible dose, 0.2 to 0.6 mg per level. Similarly, the use of BMP in ALIF also enhanced the rate of fusion compared with control groups (91% vs 79%); indeed, there is the most evidence to support the use of BMP for ALIFs. However, there is a higher rate of complications when using BMP in ALIFs, including a higher rate of retrograde ejaculation. With regard to TLIFs, the use of BMP had minimal effect with regard to fusion rates when compared with controls. The rate of adverse events, especially of postsurgical rates of radiculopathy, increased in the BMP groups. Finally, for posterolateral lumbar spinal fusions, BMP was shown to enhance fusion with minimal side effects.

These data largely reflect the manner in which BMP is used: off-label use for fusions in ALIFs, ACDFs, and posterior lumbar spinal fusions. The risk-benefit profile for these usages appears to be low, and the enhanced rate of fusion is clearly evident.

SUMMARY

It is the authors' opinion that BMP provides excellent enhancement of fusion in many spinal surgeries. However, BMP should be a cautionary tale about the use of industry-sponsored research, perceived conflicts of interest, and holding the field of spinal surgery to the highest academic scrutiny and ethical standards. In the case of BMP, not having a transparent base of literature as it was approved led to delays in allowing this superior technology to help patients.

ACKNOWLEDGMENTS

The authors thank the staff at San Francisco General Hospital for their help throughout the data collection process.

REFERENCES

1. Urist MR. Bone: formation by autoinduction. Science 1965;150:893–9.
2. Martin GJ, Boden SD, Marone MA, et al. Posterolateral intertransverse process spinal arthrodesis with rhBMP-2 in a nonhuman primate: important lessons learned regarding dose, carrier, and safety. J Spinal Disord 1999;12:179–86.
3. Boden SD, Zdeblick TA, Sandhu HS, et al. The use of rhBMP-2 in interbody fusion cages. Definitive evidence of osteoinduction in humans: a preliminary report. Spine 2000;25:376–81.
4. Boden SD, Kang J, Sandhu H, et al. Use of recombinant human bone morphogenetic protein-2 to achieve posterolateral lumbar spine fusion in humans: a prospective, randomized clinical pilot trial: 2002 Volvo Award in clinical studies. Spine 2002; 27:2662–73.
5. Burkus JK, Gornet MF, Dickman CA, et al. Anterior lumbar interbody fusion using rhBMP-2 with tapered interbody cages. J Spinal Disord Tech 2002;15: 337–49.
6. Baskin DS, Ryan P, Sonntag V, et al. A prospective, randomized, controlled cervical fusion study using recombinant human bone morphogenetic protein-2 with the CORNERSTONE-SR allograft ring and the ATLANTIS. Spine (Phila Pa 1976) 2003;28(12): 1219–24.
7. Haid RW, Branch CL, Alexander JT, et al. Posterior lumbar interbody fusion using recombinant human bone morphogenetic protein type 2 with cylindrical interbody cages. Spine J 2004;4:527–38 [discussion: 538–9].
8. Dimar JR, Glassman SD, Burkus KJ, et al. Clinical outcomes and fusion success at 2 years of single-level instrumented posterolateral fusions with recombinant human bone morphogenetic protein-2/ compression resistant matrix versus iliac crest bone graft. Spine 2006;31:2534–9.
9. Dimar JR, Glassman SD, Burkus JK, et al. Clinical and radiographic analysis of an optimized rhBMP-2 formulation as an autograft replacement in posterolateral lumbar spine arthrodesis. J Bone Joint Surg Am 2009;91:1377–86.
10. Carragee EJ, Bono CM, Scuderi GJ. Pseudomorbidity in iliac crest bone graft harvesting: the rise of rhBMP-2 in shortsegmentposterior lumbar fusion. Spine J 2009;9:873–9.
11. Hofstetter, Christoph P, Anna HS, et al. Exploratory meta-analysis on dose-related efficacy and morbidity of bone morphogenetic protein in spinal arthrodesis surgery. Journal of Neurosurgery Spine 2016; 457–75.
12. Kuklo TR, Groth AT, Anderson RC, et al. Recombinant human bone morphogenetic protein-2 for grade III open segmental tibial fractures from combat injuries in Iraq. J Bone Joint Surgery 2008; 90(8):1068–72.
13. Scott J. Withdrawal of Paper: Recombinant human bone morphogenetic protein-2 for grade III open segmental tibial fractures from combat injuries in Iraq. J Bone Joint Surgery 2009;91(3):285–6.

Lumbar Radiculopathy in the Setting of Degenerative Scoliosis
MIS Decompression and Limited Correction are Better Options

Ricardo B. Fontes, MD, PhD*, Richard G. Fessler, MD, PhD

KEYWORDS

- Scoliosis • Kyphosis • Intervertebral disc degeneration • Minimally invasive surgery

KEY POINTS

- Corrective surgery for adult spinal deformity is known to be effective but carries elevated potential morbidity whether through an open or minimally invasive technique.
- Stiffness is an adverse effect of long thoracolumbar fusions and may be particularly bothersome for younger and more active patients.
- In certain subgroups such as the very active or very sick, limited decompression or fusion in adult spinal deformity may be an attractive treatment option with fewer complications and potential shorter durability.

INTRODUCTION

The development of surgical treatments for adult degenerative deformity has been one of the biggest advances in spine surgery in the past 20 years. This has been enabled by advances in the understanding of the pathophysiology of disc degeneration and behavior of the human spine during normal and abnormal aging coupled with improvements in implant engineering, anesthetic, critical care, and surgical techniques. This has resulted in a considerable body of evidence based on individual and group case series and large, multicenter retrospective databases supporting the notion that surgery for lumbar adult spinal deformity (ASD) is safe, clinically effective, durable, and even cost-effective in most patients.[1] It has also become equally evident that treatment of ASD is associated with larger and costlier procedures with complication rates that approach 70% and mortality rates in experienced hands of around 1%.[2] There are emerging correction techniques that utilize a combination of multiple minimally invasive techniques (MIS). While the resulting combined result can hardly be called minimally invasive, it does offer a considerable decrease in morbidity to rates approaching 30% but also with reoperation rates ranging from 11% to 28%.[3–6] There is a subgroup of patients in whom a small procedure not addressing the global deformity may be advantageous either as a temporary or definitive treatment. This article's objective is to report who these patients are in the authors' deformity practice, their rationale for not

Disclosure: R.B.V. Fontes would like to report consultant work for Stryker Spine and Medtronic, none of which relates to the subject of this article.
Department of Neurosurgery, Rush University Medical Center, 1725 W Harrison, Suite 855, Chicago, IL 60612, USA
* Corresponding author.
E-mail address: Ricardo_fontes@rush.edu

neurosurgery.theclinics.com

offering deformity correction to these patients, and to discuss the data available to support this practice.

CASE EXAMPLE

A 75-year-old woman presents with long-standing back and right leg pain. She has rheumatoid arthritis and is on maintenance oral steroids. She has a clinical diagnosis of osteoporosis due to a prior L5 vertebral compression fracture and was treated 5 years ago with alendronate therapy. On examination, she is overall balanced from an alignment standpoint. She has no neck or arm pain, and her gait is normal, but reflexes are slightly increased in all 4 extremities. She has typical rheumatoid changes in both her hands. Her pain localizes to typical bilateral L5 radiculopathies and has been refractory to physical therapy, activity modification, analgesics and neuropathic pain modulators, and an L4-5 epidural steroid injection. She had undergone prior L5-S1 laminectomy 15 years prior. Her films show a baseline typical adolescent scoliosis curve with superimposed lumbar degenerative features with overall good alignment (SVA = −10 mm, and C7-CSVL is zero) (**Fig. 1**). Because of increased reflexes found on examination, a cervical MRI was ordered, which showed a number of segmentation congenital defects along with superimposed arthritic changes with cord compression (**Fig. 2**). Her lumbar MRI shows diffuse disc degeneration with varying degrees of foraminal and lateral recess stenosis and a complete canal block at L5-S1 (**Fig. 3**).

This patient adamantly refused a major anterior–posterior cervical reconstruction for her mild cervical myelopathy and was obviously

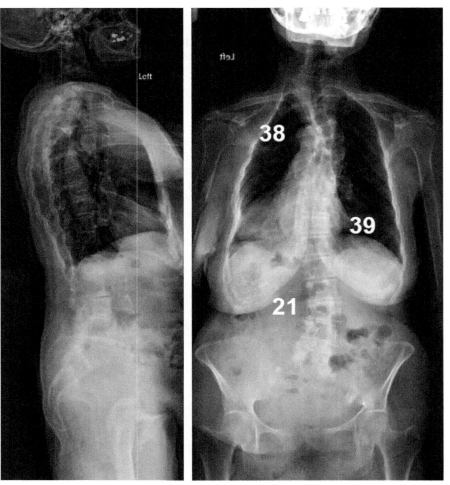

Fig. 1. 75-year-old with adolescent-type coronal curves and superimposed degenerative deformity with balanced parameters (SVA = −10 mm, PI 64°, PT 27° and lumbar lordosis 38°). PI, pelvic incidence; PT, pelvic tilt.

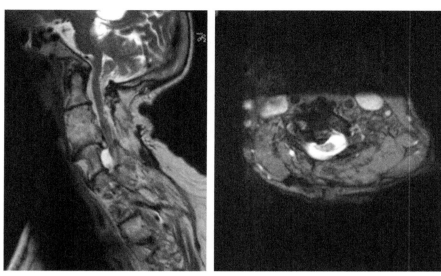

Fig. 2. Cervical MRI demonstrating segmentation defects and spinal cord compression at C4-5 with myelomalacia.

considered elevated risk for either open or MIS correction of her deformity. A compromise was reached, and awake L4-5 and L5-S1 minimally invasive laminectomies under spinal block and local anesthesia was offered; this allowed the patient to position herself in a prone position and protect her neck. She underwent a 75-minute procedure with minimal discomfort and was discharged home the following day. Her back and leg Visual Analog Scale (VAS) scores dropped from 8 of 10 to 5 of 10 and 1 of 10, respectively, and Oswestry Disability Index (ODI) from 44 to 9 at 6 months postoperatively. Postoperative MRI shows effective lateral recess decompression at L5-S1 (**Fig. 4**).

TREATMENT RATIONALE AND DISCUSSION

Literature supporting a limited, focal treatment in the setting of ASD is sparse. The first relatively obvious indication is in patients too sick or too elderly to undergo a full correction population, as shown in the case example. However, the authors have also identified a group of high-functioning, young patients who present with predominantly limb pain who are not willing to undergo a long fusion and its consequences. Stiffness as a consequence of a long fusion may be a limitation for sports and more demanding daily activities. Hart and colleagues[7] developed the Lumbar Stiffness Disability Index to evaluate this problem. They

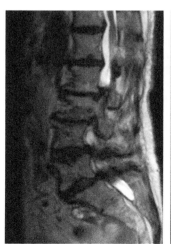
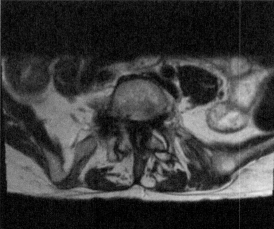

Fig. 3. Lumbar MRI with multilevel disc degeneration and severe foraminal stenosis, along with very severe lateral recess stenosis at L5-S1 (axial view).

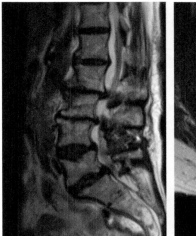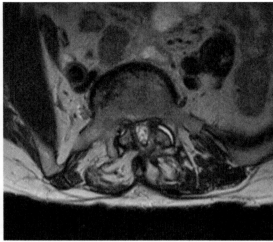

Fig. 4. MRI 6 months after surgery with efficient decompression. Patient is doing very well, with minimal pain and increased ambulation distance 12-fold.

demonstrated that a single-level fusion may actually improve mobility because of its effects in alleviating pain and has minimal effects on range of motion (ROM), but a 3-level fusion already leads to consistent perception of loss of ROM, which is worse with a 5-level fusion.[8] This impact is somewhat mitigated in ASD as these patients already have significant limitation in ROM preoperatively, but invariably there is a significant decrease in residual mobility after the fusion.[9,10] Patients undergoing instrumented fusion with an uppermost instrumented vertebra (UIV) in the thoracolumbar region may expect difficulties initially in bathing and dressing the lower half of their bodies, and those undergoing even longer fusions to the upper thoracic area may expect additional difficulty in performing personal hygiene after toileting.[10,11] The caudal level does not seem to be as important, and a lower instrumented vertebra (LIV) at L5 or S1 seems to not differ in terms of perceived stiffness.[10] These are important points to discuss with patients undergoing treatment for ASD and easily explain why patients in the fifth or sixth decade may be unhappier as their expectations regarding daily activities may be more stringent. The authors have found that these patients may sometimes rather deal with some amount of residual back pain and delay an eventual long fusion into the seventh decade, rather than pay the price of restricted mobility upfront.

Few authors have analyzed the impact of limited decompression or fusion in the setting of ASD. Madhavan and colleagues[12] analyzed the role of endoscopic foraminotomy in well-balanced patients with coronal curves between 10° and 20° and reported satisfactory improvements in VAS

scores postoperatively. Transfeldt and colleagues[13] compared decompression alone, decompression and limited fusion, and complete decompression and fusion in patients with ASD. These groups differed significantly in their complication rates (56% for the full fusion group vs 10% for decompression alone). Clinical improvement was evident in all 3 groups, with the biggest improvements in ODI in the decompression and limited fusion groups and the greatest satisfaction scores in the full-fusion group. It is worthwhile noting that the decompression alone group had the oldest patients and had the most limited follow-up, which may not account for progression of ASD. Kleinstueck and colleagues[14] showed in a retrospective study that patients undergoing decompression or a short-segment fusion for ASD had lower complication rates and outcome measures just slightly inferior to those undergoing a long fusion. The caveat to this study is that these are not randomized patients but rather patients specifically selected to undergo decompression only if they were sicker and/or had predominantly leg and not back pain. Cho and colleagues[15] also showed good results with short-segment fusion if ASD patients were balanced and had small (10°–20°) coronal Cobb angles, particularly if there was a focal deformity (eg, spondylolisthesis) with the corrected area. Kasliwal and colleagues[16] have shown that a prior arthrodesis does not predispose to worse outcome when undergoing the large procedure for ASD, only that its durability may be compromised. It is worth noting, however, that this study started with patients undergoing the full correction and thus corresponded to eventual failures of the short segment fusion; persistent successes may never be captured by these studies utilizing the large ASD databases.

SUMMARY

An aggressive, "have-curve-will-fuse" strategy in ASD is by no means correct in every situation. Although correction of ASD particularly with sagittal plane imbalance is proven to be effective and durable, it carries considerable significant perioperative risks and morbidity in terms of loss of ROM. Limited surgical intervention through a simple decompression or limited fusion may be advantageous in selected, sagittally balanced subgroups such as the very sick, as long as the patient and treatment team understand results may not be durable if there is progression of the deformity. It may also be a good strategy for very active patients wishing to delay full correction of deformity and its inherent side effect of rigidity and does not result in any difficulty later when performing the longer correction for ASD.

REFERENCES

1. Scheer JK, Hostin R, Robinson C, et al. Operative management of adult spinal deformity results in significant increases in QALYs gained compared to non-operative management: analysis of 479 patients with minimum 2-year follow-up. Spine 2016. [Epub ahead of print].

2. Smith JS, Klineberg E, Lafage V, et al. Prospective multicenter assessment of perioperative and minimum 2-year postoperative complication rates associated with adult spinal deformity surgery. J Neurosurg Spine 2016;25(1):1–14.

3. Hamilton DK, Kanter AS, Bolinger BD, et al. Reoperation rates in minimally invasive, hybrid and open surgical treatment for adult spinal deformity with minimum 2-year follow-up. Eur Spine J 2016;25(8): 2605–11.

4. Park P, Wang MY, Lafage V, et al. Comparison of two minimally invasive surgery strategies to treat adult spinal deformity. J Neurosurg Spine 2015;22(4): 374–80.

5. Uribe JS, Deukmedjian AR, Mummaneni PV, et al. Complications in adult spinal deformity surgery: an analysis of minimally invasive, hybrid, and open surgical techniques. Neurosurg Focus 2014;36(5):E15.

6. Yen C-P, Mosley YI, Uribe JS. Role of minimally invasive surgery for adult spinal deformity in preventing complications. Curr Rev Musculoskelet Med 2016; 9(3):309–15.

7. Hart RA, Gundle KR, Pro SL, et al. Lumbar stiffness disability index: pilot testing of consistency, reliability, and validity. Spine J 2013;13(2):157–61.

8. Hart RA, Marshall LM, Hiratzka SL, et al. Functional limitations due to stiffness as a collateral impact of instrumented arthrodesis of the lumbar spine. Spine 2014;39(24):E1468–74.

9. Daniels AH, Smith JS, Hiratzka J, et al. Functional limitations due to lumbar stiffness in adults with and without spinal deformity. Spine 2015;40(20): 1599–604.

10. Daniels AH, Koller H, Hiratzka SL, et al. Selecting caudal fusion levels: 2 year functional and stiffness outcomes with matched pairs analysis in multilevel fusion to L5 versus S1. Eur Spine J 2016. [Epub ahead of print].

11. Sciubba DM, Scheer JK, Smith JS, et al. Which daily functions are most affected by stiffness following total lumbar fusion: comparison of upper thoracic and thoracolumbar proximal endpoints. Spine 2015; 40(17):1338–44.

12. Madhavan K, Chieng LO, McGrath L, et al. Early experience with endoscopic foraminotomy in patients with moderate degenerative deformity. Neurosurg Focus 2016;40(2):E6.

13. Transfeldt EE, Topp R, Mehbod AA, et al. Surgical outcomes of decompression, decompression with limited fusion, and decompression with full curve fusion for degenerative scoliosis with radiculopathy. Spine 2010;35(20):1872–5.

14. Kleinstueck FS, Fekete TF, Jeszenszky D, et al. Adult degenerative scoliosis: comparison of patient-rated outcome after three different surgical treatments. Eur Spine J 2016;25(8):2649–56.

15. Cho K-J, Suk S-I, Park S-R, et al. Short fusion versus long fusion for degenerative lumbar scoliosis. Eur Spine J 2008;17(5):650–6.

16. Kasliwal MK, Smith JS, Shaffrey CI, et al. Does prior short-segment surgery for adult scoliosis impact perioperative complication rates and clinical outcome among patients undergoing scoliosis correction? J Neurosurg Spine 2012;17(2):128–33.

The Case for Deformity Correction in the Management of Radiculopathy with Concurrent Spinal Deformity

CrossMark

Sigurd Berven, MD*, Anthony DiGiorgio, DO

KEYWORDS

- Adult spinal deformity • Treatment strategies • Decompression alone
- Decompression with limited fusion • Multilevel fusion • Appropriate use criteria • Clinical outcomes

KEY POINTS

- Adult spinal deformity may present with a spectrum of clinical presentations, including radiculopathy, back pain, and deformity.
- The appropriate management of symptomatic adult deformity is the strategy that optimizes the clinical outcome of care while limiting the risk and costs of care.
- In the setting of spinal deformity that contributes to the clinical presentation of radiculopathy, decompression alone presents significant risk for poor outcomes, including revision surgery, due to inadequate creation of space for the neural elements, inadequate realignment of the spine, and progression of deformity.
- Decompression with limited fusion is most appropriate for patients with focal radicular pain and deformity that is stable, with good global sagittal and coronal alignment.
- Decompression with more extensive fusion and realignment of the spine is most appropriate for patients with focal radicular pain, and deformity that is progressive or that involves global malalignment in the sagittal or coronal planes.

INTRODUCTION

Adult spinal deformity is a common and important pathologic condition affecting the spinal column. The impact of spinal deformity on the health status of affected patients is significant, It affects domains of health, including pain, function, mental health, and self-image.[1,2] The burden of disease that is encompassed by spinal deformity may be measured by both the prevalence of the disorder, and the impact of the disorder on affected patients.[3] The prevalence of deformity in the aging spine is common, and spinal deformity contributes to the clinical presentation of back pain in most women older than age 60 years.[4,5] The impact of deformity on health-related quality of life is significant. Patients presenting with symptomatic spinal deformity self-report their health status preference as significantly worse than other common medical conditions, including cardiopulmonary disease, mental health disorders, and other musculoskeletal disorders.[6,7] An evidence-based approach to the appropriate management of deformity is

Department of Orthopaedic Surgery, UC San Francisco, 500 Parnassus Avenue, MU320W, San Francisco, CA 94143-0728, USA
* Corresponding author.
E-mail address: Sigurd.Berven@ucsf.edu

Neurosurg Clin N Am 28 (2017) 341–347
http://dx.doi.org/10.1016/j.nec.2017.03.002
1042-3680/17/© 2017 Elsevier Inc. All rights reserved.

important because of the prevalence, impact, and burden of adult deformity. The management of patients with radiculopathy and adult deformity is characterized by significant variability, with options encompassing decompression alone, decompression with a limited fusion, and decompression with a multilevel fusion for realignment of the spine. This article reviews the spectrum of surgical approaches for the management of symptomatic lumbar deformity with radiculopathy and provides guidance for an evidence-based approach to when less invasive procedures may be appropriate and when more invasive procedures, including deformity correction, are appropriate.

The Relationship Between Deformity and Symptomatic Radiculopathy

Spinal deformity encompasses a spectrum of malalignments of the spine, including segmental, regional, and global deformity. There is a significant correlation between deformity of the spine and health status, with significant compromise of pain, function, and self-image associated with global, regional, and segmental malalignment.[8,9]

Adult spinal deformity commonly presents with both back pain and radicular symptoms.[10–12] The cause of low back pain in adult spinal deformity is multifactorial and related to symptomatic degeneration of the functional motion segment, asymmetric loading of the spinal column, and soft tissue imbalances. Musculoligamentous strain, facet arthropathy, disc degeneration, and compression of neural elements can all contribute to axial back pain.[13] Disc degeneration and loss of height causes a loss of lordosis, whereas asymmetric degeneration leads to a scoliotic curvature.[14] Therefore, advanced degenerative scoliosis is characterized by both lumbar hypolordosis and coronal deformity, including rotational subluxation. The low back pain in adult spinal deformity tends to correlate with a loss of lumbar lordosis,[15] whereas the presence of a scoliotic curve itself is not sufficient to cause pain but can contribute to it in the presence of symptomatic degeneration.[5]

Neural symptoms are an important part of the clinical presentation of adult deformity, and an important reason that patients choose to pursue operative care for deformity.[16] Deformity of the spine contributes directly to neural compression and symptoms attributable to compression of neural structures, commonly radiculopathy or neurogenic claudication.[10–13,17] A scoliotic curve can lead to central stenosis, which is greatest at the apex.[11] Nerve roots can be compressed on either side of a curve. Roots on the concave side are

compressed by foraminal or extraforaminal stenosis. Foraminal stenosis may be especially severe at the concavity where adjacent pedicles are in close proximity. An adequate decompression requires removal of most or all of the facet joint and realignment of the spine to create foraminal volume. Roots on the convex side are more affected by stenosis in the lateral recess and an increase in tension of the exiting roots on the side of the convexity.[18] Olisthesis decreases dural sac cross-sectional diameter, leading to central canal stenosis and claudication. Disc bulging, reactive hypertrophy of the ligamentum flavum, and bony overgrowth exacerbate the stenosis centrally, foraminally, and in the lateral recess.[19] Treatment of symptomatic radiculopathy often requires realignment of the spine for adequate decompression of the neural elements. A decompression alone with facet preservation and unchanged alignment of the spine is often inadequate for neural decompression.

VARIABILITY IN APPROACHES TO CARE

The management of lumbar radiculopathy in the setting of spinal deformity is characterized by significant variability. The presence of variability is clear evidence of the absence of an evidence-based approach to care. The appropriate management of adult degenerative scoliosis is the treatment that leads to the most reliable improvement of health-related quality of life while limiting the risks of complications and harm.[20] In a value-based health care economy, the cost of care is also an important consideration. Appropriate care is the strategy that optimizes the clinical outcome while minimizing both risk and costs of care.[21] An evidence-based approach to the management of symptomatic radiculopathy with spinal deformity may include decompression alone, decompression with limited fusion, or decompression with extensive realignment of the spine. The most appropriate treatment requires an understanding of the type of deformity, curve characteristics, and alignment of the spine.

DECOMPRESSION ALONE

Decompression procedures have relatively low costs and complication rates.[22] When performed in a patient with a stable spine, a simple decompression has been shown to be cost-effective.[23] However, the removal of bony elements and soft tissue disruption required for decompressive procedures have the potential to exacerbate existing deformity. A classic study by Herkowitz and colleagues[24] demonstrates significantly improved outcomes in patients with spondylolisthesis treated with posterolateral fusion compared with decompression alone. More recently, Houten and Nasser[25] reported rapid progression of deformity with limited decompression in the setting of scoliosis.[24] Several investigators have reported high rates of progressive deformity and failure of surgery in patients with deformity and symptomatic stenosis.[26–28]

The presence of pre-existing instability increases the chances that a decompression will fail, whereas a stable deformity indicates a decompression alone may be appropriate. The stable spine is the spine that can withstand physiologic loads without risk of progressive deformity, segmental translation, or compromise of the neural elements. Stability can be determined by dynamic radiographs, including flexion and extension views, and radiographic assessments, including the presence of bridging osteophytes.

The effect of decompression alone on the spine with segmental olisthesis, rotatory subluxation, or scoliosis is to further compromise segmental stability without improving segmental alignment of the spine. A recent randomized trial by Forsth and colleagues[29] showed equivocal outcomes and reoperation rates in subjects treated with simple decompression versus decompression and fusion for lumbar stenosis with spondylolisthesis. However, they did not evaluate stability in their trial. A series by Modhia and colleagues[30] showed that revision surgery rates were similar in subjects undergoing decompression versus decompression with fusion. Cases involving instability were excluded and preoperative deformity was not recorded.

A series by Katz and colleagues[31] retrospectively reviewed 7-year to 10-year follow-up data for spinal stenosis treated with decompression. They found that 23% of subjects required a revision. However, they did not measure preoperative deformity parameters or identify risk factors for reoperation. At final follow-up, 33% of subjects continued to have severe back pain and 76% were satisfied with their outcome.

A retrospective study by Hosogane and colleagues[32] reviewed 50 subjects who had a coronal deformity 1 year after decompression surgery. Ten percent of subjects required revision surgery at 33-month follow-up but none of the indications were related to deformity progression. Of the parameters to predict curve progression, they found that osteophyte formation on the curve concavity was the only factor that was protective. Hansraj and colleagues[33] reviewed 50 elderly subjects with deformity and symptomatic stenosis who were treated with decompression alone. Their

cohort had a Cobb angle less than 20° and no segmental translation or instability, with only 5% undergoing revision over 5 years. Decompression alone may be appropriate for the group of patients who have smaller curves (<20°); segmental stability, including bridging osteophytes; and radiculopathy that does not require realignment of the spine for adequate decompression.

DECOMPRESSION WITH LIMITED FUSION

Lumbar decompression with limited fusion enables the surgeon to widely decompress the neural elements, including complete facetectomy, and to realign the spine for indirect neural decompression. Decompression with a limited fusion may be a cost-effective and durable procedure for cases with symptomatic radiculopathy and deformity.[34–36] Significant variability among surgeons remains in the specifics on instrumentation, interbody graft, and circumferential arthrodesis. Instrumentation and approach are among the most significant determinants of the cost of these procedures.[37] Overall, however, operative interventions provide superior value for treating spinal disorders with associated nerve compression and instability, as demonstrated in a systematic review by Indrakanti and colleagues[38] comparing operative with nonoperative interventions.

The lower lumbar spine, exposed to higher mechanical stress, is a common source of pain from facet arthropathy and spinal stenosis. Pain and neural compression can additionally arise from fractional curves in this area.[12] Even in the presence of spinal deformity, if overall global alignment remains normal, a limited fusion of the symptomatic curve can improve pain without incurring the risk and costs of an extensive deformity correction (**Fig. 1**). Figure 1 demonstrates a decompression with limited fusion for a patient with adult degenerative scoliosis and radicular pain related to the concavity of the deformity.

A recent randomized trial by Ghogawala and colleagues[36] showed significantly higher quality of life scores in subjects undergoing fusion for spondylolisthesis when compared with decompression alone. They also showed a lower rate of revision surgery in the fusion group at 4 years. Additionally, the use of instrumentation increases the rates of fusion and improves outcomes when compared with noninstrumented arthrodesis.[39–41]

Similarly, circumferential fusion costs more up front but may be justified by saving money over time. Han and colleagues[42] performed a meta-analysis examining prospective trials that compared circumferential fusion to posterior fusion alone. They found that the circumferential

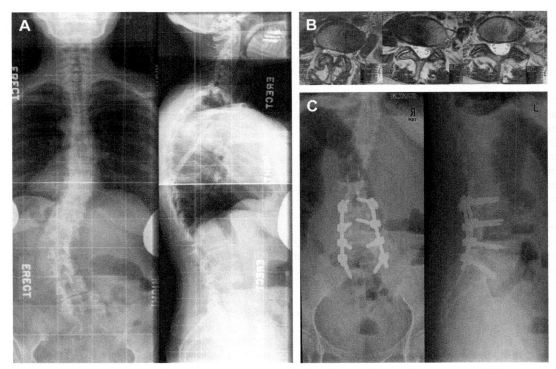

Fig. 1. A 68-year-old woman with longstanding lumbar scoliosis without evidence of progression. (*A*) Preoperative AP and Lateral images. Patient with limited left L4 and L5 radicular pain that has been persistent despite 2 prior decompressive procedures. (*B*) MRI axial images at L3-4, L4-5 and L5-S1. (*C*) Post-operative AP and Lateral images. Patient was treated with a limited decompression and fusion from L3 to S1 with correction of the fractional curve and both direct and indirect decompression of the concave stenosis at L4-5 and L5-S1. Patient has had no recurrence of radicular pain at more than 5-year follow-up.

fusions had more complications and blood loss but better long-term outcomes and fewer reoperations. Soegaard and colleagues[43] found a cost savings of nearly $50,000 per quality-adjusted life year with similarly decreased reoperations and improved outcomes.

The question of the length of the fusion remains unanswered. Longer fusions, although including more of the deformity and preventing proximal progression, can lead to longer operating times, greater complications, proximal junctional kyphosis, and pseudoarthrosis. Cho and colleagues[44] reported outcomes on 50 subjects who underwent a long or short fusion. The long fusion group had slightly higher preoperative Cobb angle and better postoperative coronal correction. There was no statistically significant difference in sagittal correction. None of their subjects underwent a 3-column osteotomy.

DECOMPRESSION WITH EXTENSIVE FUSION

Correction of adult spinal deformity with the goal of re-establishing global realignment typically requires a complex surgical reconstruction. These extensive procedures often involve spinal osteotomies and are associated with increased complications and cost. This is exacerbated by a high prevalence of comorbidities in this patient population. It has yet to be determined where they fit in with a value-based health care system because, although the clinical improvement may be significant in most cases, the costs and complications are high.

Sagittal alignment is the most significant predictor of poor health status in adults with spinal deformity.[45] Restoration of sagittal alignment is the primary goal of deformity correction surgery. The impact of deformity on health status has been classified by Schwab and colleagues.[5] Parameters used to determine imbalance are the sagittal vertical axis, pelvic tilt, and T1 pelvic angle. Correcting these parameters involves restoration of anterior column height, often requiring combined anterior and posterior procedures, and extensive spine osteotomies. Unfortunately, patients that present with symptomatic deformity and sagittal plane imbalance are unlikely to improve without restoring lumbar lordosis that matches the pelvic incidence, and correcting the pelvic tilt and sagittal vertical axis deviation. Limited decompressions and decompression with limited fusion are not procedures that can lead to a reliable improvement of global malalignment of the spine.

Patients treated with extensive spinal reconstructions for symptomatic deformity have shown significant improvement on self-reported outcomes, despite the high complication rates. Daubs and colleagues[46] had major complications in 20% of subjects older than 60 years and an overall complication rate of 37% in the same cohort. Despite this, subjects reported improved outcomes overall.

Even patients older than the age of 75 years show more improvement with operative correction of spinal deformity when compared with nonoperative management. Sciubba and colleagues[47] showed significantly improved health-related quality of life measures in subjects in the operative cohort. This was despite a complication rate of 75%. These data can be useful in counseling patients and families when considering surgical options.

A retrospective review by Kleinstueck and colleagues[48] recently compared the 3 approaches of decompression alone, decompression with limited fusion, and decompression with extensive reconstruction of the spine. Operative time, blood loss, and complication rates all increased with the more extensive approaches. However, all 3 groups showed equivalent improvements in self-reported outcomes (good outcomes in 69%, 74%, and 76%, respectively). The investigators concluded that appropriate patient selection and choice of the appropriate intervention for each patient is the determinant of good outcomes. No predictors of bad outcomes were identified.

SUMMARY

The management of patients with symptomatic radiculopathy with concurrent spinal deformity is characterized by significant variability between providers who care for patients with spinal disorders. Deformity of the spine contributes directly to axial and radicular pain patterns, and realignment of the spine is often required for an adequate direct and indirect decompression of the neural elements. Decompression alone is inappropriate for patients with segmental instability of the spine, progressive deformity, global sagittal malalignment of the spine, or radiculopathy due to foraminal narrowing at the concavity of a deformity. Decompression with limited fusion may be appropriate in patients with focal segmental instability and global alignment of the spine. Decompression with a limited fusion is especially useful in the patient with a deformity that is not progressive and that is globally well-aligned, as well as in cases in which radicular symptoms are primarily at the concavity of the fractional curve from L4 to S1. The patient with symptomatic radiculopathy and deformity that involves progression and global malalignment requires a more extensive reconstruction of the spine with restoration of segmental, regional, and global alignment for a reliable improvement of health-related quality of life. Understanding curve characteristics, including segmental stability and progression, the pathoanatomy or nerve compression, and global alignment of the spine, is important for informed decision-making on the appropriate approach to surgical management of patients with symptomatic radiculopathy and spinal deformity.

REFERENCES

1. Berven S, Deviren V, Demir-Deviren S, et al. Studies in the modified Scoliosis Research Society outcomes instrument in adults: validation, reliability, and discriminatory capacity. Spine (Phila Pa 1976) 2003;28(18):2164–9 [discussion: 2169].

2. Crawford CH 3rd, Glassman SD, Bridwell KH, et al. The minimum clinically important difference in SRS-22R total score, appearance, activity and pain domains after surgical treatment of adult spinal deformity. Spine (Phila Pa 1976) 2015;40(6):377–81.

3. In scientific opportunities and public needs: improving priority setting and public input at the national institutes of health. Washington (DC): National Academy Press; 1998.

4. Healey JH, Lane JM. Structural scoliosis in osteoporotic women. Clin Orthop Relat Res 1985;(195):216–23.

5. Schwab F, Dubey A, Gamez L, et al. Adult scoliosis: prevalence, SF-36, and nutritional parameters in an elderly volunteer population. Spine (Phila Pa 1976) 2005;30(9):1082–5.

6. Pellise F, Vila-Casademunt A, Ferrer M, et al. Impact on health related quality of life of adult spinal deformity (ASD) compared with other chronic conditions. Eur Spine J 2015;24(1):3–11.

7. Bess S, Line B, Fu KM, et al. the health impact of symptomatic adult spinal deformity: comparison of deformity types to United States population norms and chronic diseases. Spine (Phila Pa 1976) 2016; 41(3):224–33.

8. Schwab F, Farcy JP, Bridwell K, et al. A clinical impact classification of scoliosis in the adult. Spine (Phila Pa 1976) 2006;31(18):2109–14.

9. Bess S, Schwab F, Lafage V, et al. Classifications for adult spinal deformity and use of the Scoliosis Research Society-Schwab adult spinal deformity

classification. Neurosurg Clin N Am 2013;24(2):185–93.

10. Heary RF, Kumar S, Bono CM. Decision making in adult deformity. Neurosurgery 2008;63(3 Suppl): 69–77.

11. Pritchett JW, Bortel DT. Degenerative symptomatic lumbar scoliosis. Spine (Phila Pa 1976) 1993;18(6): 700–3.

12. Liu W, Chen XS, Jia LS, et al. The clinical features and surgical treatment of degenerative lumbar scoliosis: a review of 112 patients. Orthop Surg 2009; 1(3):176–83.

13. Bradford DS, Tay BK, Hu SS. Adult scoliosis: surgical indications, operative management, complications, and outcomes. Spine (Phila Pa 1976) 1999; 24(24):2617–29.

14. Murata Y, Takahashi K, Hanaoka E, et al. Changes in scoliotic curvature and lordotic angle during the early phase of degenerative lumbar scoliosis. Spine (Phila Pa 1976) 2002;27(20):2268–73.

15. Tsuji T, Matsuyama Y, Sato K, et al. Epidemiology of low back pain in the elderly: correlation with lumbar lordosis. J Orthop Sci 2001;6(4):307–11.

16. Pekmezci M, Berven SH, Hu SS, et al. The factors that play a role in the decision-making process of adult deformity patients. Spine (Phila Pa 1976) 2009;34(8):813–7.

17. Glassman SD, Schwab FJ, Bridwell KH, et al. The selection of operative versus nonoperative treatment in patients with adult scoliosis. Spine (Phila Pa 1976) 2007;32(1):93–7.

18. Liu H, Ishihara H, Kanamori M, et al. Characteristics of nerve root compression caused by degenerative lumbar spinal stenosis with scoliosis. Spine J 2003; 3(6):524–9.

19. Ploumis A, Transfeldt EE, Gilbert TJ Jr, et al. Degenerative lumbar scoliosis: radiographic correlation of lateral rotatory olisthesis with neural canal dimensions. Spine (Phila Pa 1976) 2006;31(20):2353–8.

20. Chen PG, Daubs MD, Berven S, et al. Surgery for degenerative lumbar scoliosis: the development of appropriateness criteria. Spine (Phila Pa 1976) 2016;41(10):910–8.

21. Porter ME, Teisberg EO. Redefining health care: creating value-based competition on results. Boston: Harvard Business School Press; 2006. p. xvii, 506.

22. Deyo RA, Mirza SK, Martin BI, et al. Trends, major medical complications, and charges associated with surgery for lumbar spinal stenosis in older adults. JAMA 2010;303(13):1259–65.

23. Tosteson AN, Lurie JD, Tosteson TD, et al. Surgical treatment of spinal stenosis with and without degenerative spondylolisthesis: cost-effectiveness after 2 years. Ann Intern Med 2008;149(12):845–53.

24. Herkowitz HN, Kurz LT. Degenerative lumbar spondylolisthesis with spinal stenosis. A prospective study comparing decompression with decompression and intertransverse process arthrodesis. J Bone Joint Surg Am 1991;73(6):802–8.

25. Houten JK, Nasser R. Symptomatic progression of degenerative scoliosis after decompression and limited fusion surgery for lumbar spinal stenosis. J Clin Neurosci 2013;20(4):613–5.

26. Frazier DD, Lipson SJ, Fossel AH, et al. Associations between spinal deformity and outcomes after decompression for spinal stenosis. Spine (Phila Pa 1976) 1997;22(17):2025–9.

27. Aebi M. The adult scoliosis. Eur Spine J 2005; 14(10):925–48.

28. Simmons ED. Surgical treatment of patients with lumbar spinal stenosis with associated scoliosis. Clin Orthop Relat Res 2001;(384):45–53.

29. Forsth P, Ólafsson G, Carlsson T, et al. A randomized, controlled trial of fusion surgery for lumbar spinal stenosis. N Engl J Med 2016; 374(15):1413–23.

30. Modhia U, Takemoto S, Braid-Forbes MJ, et al. Readmission rates after decompression surgery in patients with lumbar spinal stenosis among Medicare beneficiaries. Spine (Phila Pa 1976) 2013;38(7):591–6.

31. Katz JN, Lipson SJ, Chang LC, et al. Seven- to 10-year outcome of decompressive surgery for degenerative lumbar spinal stenosis. Spine (Phila Pa 1976) 1996;21(1):92–8.

32. Hosogane N, Watanabe K, Kono H, et al. Curve progression after decompression surgery in patients with mild degenerative scoliosis. J Neurosurg Spine 2013;18(4):321–6.

33. Hansraj KK, Cammisa FP Jr, O'Leary PF, et al. Decompressive surgery for typical lumbar spinal stenosis. Clin Orthop Relat Res 2001;(384):10–7.

34. Devin CJ, Chotai S, Parker SL, et al. A cost-utility analysis of lumbar decompression with and without fusion for degenerative spine disease in the elderly. Neurosurgery 2015;77(Suppl 4): S116–24.

35. Weinstein JN, Lurie JD, Tosteson TD, et al. Surgical compared with nonoperative treatment for lumbar degenerative spondylolisthesis. Four-year results in the spine patient outcomes research trial (SPORT) randomized and observational cohorts. J Bone Joint Surg Am 2009;91(6):1295–304.

36. Ghogawala Z, Dziura J, Butler WE, et al. Laminectomy plus fusion versus laminectomy alone for lumbar spondylolisthesis. N Engl J Med 2016;374(15): 1424–34.

37. McCarthy IM, Hostin RA, Ames CP, et al. Total hospital costs of surgical treatment for adult spinal deformity: an extended follow-up study. Spine J 2014; 14(10):2326–33.

38. Indrakanti SS, Weber MH, Takemoto SK, et al. Value-based care in the management of spinal disorders: a systematic review of cost-utility analysis. Clin Orthop Relat Res 2012;470(4):1106–23.

39. Okuda S, Oda T, Miyauchi A, et al. Surgical outcomes of posterior lumbar interbody fusion in elderly patients. J Bone Joint Surg Am 2006; 88(12):2714–20.

40. Cassinelli EH, Eubanks J, Vogt M, et al. Risk factors for the development of perioperative complications in elderly patients undergoing lumbar decompression and arthrodesis for spinal stenosis: an analysis of 166 patients. Spine (Phila Pa 1976) 2007;32(2): 230–5.

41. Fischgrund JS, Mackay M, Herkowitz HN, et al. 1997 Volvo Award winner in clinical studies. Degenerative lumbar spondylolisthesis with spinal stenosis: a prospective, randomized study comparing decompressive laminectomy and arthrodesis with and without spinal instrumentation. Spine (Phila Pa 1976) 1997; 22(24):2807–12.

42. Han X, Zhu Y, Cui C, et al. A meta-analysis of circumferential fusion versus instrumented posterolateral fusion in the lumbar spine. Spine (Phila Pa 1976) 2009;34(17):E618–25.

43. Soegaard R, Bünger CE, Christiansen T, et al. Circumferential fusion is dominant over posterolateral fusion in a long-term perspective: cost-utility evaluation of a randomized controlled trial in severe, chronic low back pain. Spine (Phila Pa 1976) 2007; 32(22):2405–14.

44. Cho KJ, Suk SI, Park SR, et al. Short fusion versus long fusion for degenerative lumbar scoliosis. Eur Spine J 2008;17(5):650–6.

45. Glassman SD, Berven S, Bridwell K, et al. Correlation of radiographic parameters and clinical symptoms in adult scoliosis. Spine (Phila Pa 1976) 2005; 30(6):682–8.

46. Daubs MD, Lenke LG, Cheh G, et al. Adult spinal deformity surgery: complications and outcomes in patients over age 60. Spine (Phila Pa 1976) 2007; 32(20):2238–44.

47. Sciubba DM, Scheer JK, Yurter A, et al. Patients with spinal deformity over the age of 75: a retrospective analysis of operative versus nonoperative management. Eur Spine J 2016;25(8): 2433–41.

48. Kleinstueck FS, Fekete TF, Jeszenszky D, et al. Adult degenerative scoliosis: comparison of patient-rated outcome after three different surgical treatments. Eur Spine J 2016;25(8):2649–56.

Hemicraniectomy for Ischemic and Hemorrhagic Stroke
Facts and Controversies

Aman Gupta, MD[a,b,c], Mithun G. Sattur, MD[a,b,c],
Rami James N. Aoun, MD, MPH[a,b,c], Chandan Krishna, MD[a],
Patrick B. Bolton, MD[d], Brian W. Chong, MD, FRCP(C)[a,e],
Bart M. Demaerschalk, MD, MSc, FRCP(C)[f],
Mark K. Lyons, MD[a], Jamal McClendon Jr, MD[a],
Naresh Patel, MD[a], Ayan Sen, MD[g], Kristin Swanson, PhD[a,b],
Richard S. Zimmerman, MD[a],
Bernard R. Bendok, MD, MSCI[a,b,c,e,h,*]

KEYWORDS

- Decompressive craniectomy • Malignant infarct • Cerebellar stroke • Modified Rankin score
- Cerebral edema • Surgery for stroke

KEY POINTS

- Acute occlusion of a proximal large intracranial artery has high risk of progression to malignant infarct.
- The results of best medical management including aggressive ICU measures are dismal, with mortality of up to 80%.
- Decompressive craniectomy (DC) is demonstrated to conclusively improve mortality to around 30%.
- DC also improves the chances of good functional outcome when performed within 48 hours in patients younger than 60 years of age but should be considered beyond these circumstances on a case-by-case basis.
- Better indicators of edema progression, patient eligibility, and clinical outcome measures are urgently required for use in larger randomized controlled trials.
- DC also serves an important role in managing select patients with supratentorial spontaneous hemorrhage, and posterior fossa hemorrhage and ischemic stroke.

[a] Department of Neurological Surgery, Mayo Clinic Hospital, Mayo Clinic, 5777 East Mayo Boulevard, Phoenix, AZ 85054, USA; [b] Precision Neuro-theraputics Innovation Lab, Mayo Clinic Hospital, Mayo Clinic, 5777 East Mayo Boulevard, Phoenix, AZ 85054, USA; [c] Neurosurgery Simulation and Innovation Lab, Mayo Clinic Hospital, Mayo Clinic, 5777 East Mayo Boulevard, Phoenix, AZ 85054, USA; [d] Department of Anesthesia & Periop Med, Mayo Clinic Hospital, Mayo Clinic, 5777 East Mayo Boulevard, Phoenix, AZ 85054, USA; [e] Department of Radiology, Mayo Clinic Hospital, Mayo Clinic, 5777 East Mayo Boulevard, Phoenix, AZ 85054, USA; [f] Department of Neurology, Mayo Clinic Hospital, Mayo Clinic, 5777 East Mayo Boulevard, Phoenix, AZ 85054, USA; [g] Department of Critical Care Medicine, Mayo Clinic Hospital, Mayo Clinic, 5777 East Mayo Boulevard, Phoenix, AZ 85054, USA; [h] Department of Otolaryngology, Mayo Clinic Hospital, Mayo Clinic, 5777 East Mayo Boulevard, Phoenix, AZ 85054, USA
* Corresponding author.
E-mail address: bendok.bernard@mayo.edu

Neurosurg Clin N Am 28 (2017) 349–360
http://dx.doi.org/10.1016/j.nec.2017.02.010

INTRODUCTION

Progressive global or local intracranial mass effect is frequently encountered with large hemispheric infarcts ("malignant infarcts"[1]). The resulting increased intracranial pressure (ICP) results in the potential for worsened outcomes and dramatically increased mortality. Decompressive craniectomy (with capacious duraplasty; DC) is a highly effective procedure that is often warranted in such situations. DC for ischemic stroke has been conclusively proven to reduce mortality in large hemispheric infarcts[2] and is a powerful tool in a comprehensive neurovascular team's armamentarium. Despite the utility of DC, there are schools of thought that discourage surgery because of the biased perception that patients survive but are left with severe burdensome disability. This article discusses the available literature and demonstrates the effectiveness of DC in malignant infarction and functional outcome. Also discussed is the role of DC in posterior fossa (cerebellar) stroke and spontaneous intracerebral hematomas (ICH).

ISCHEMIC HEMISPHERIC STROKE (SUPRATENTORIAL)
Epidemiology

The prevalence of malignant ischemic stroke is reported to be between 2% and 8%[3–5] of all patients with ischemic stroke. The mortality rate of patients with malignant stroke who undergo aggressive nonoperative management is in the range of 40% to 80%.[6] Performing a DC can reduce this mortality rate to 30% (**Table 1**).

Pathophysiology of Malignant Stroke

Microscopic and cellular changes
Neuronal death in ischemia occurs through apoptosis, necrosis, and autophagy.[7] Briefly, cellular events begin with deprivation of glucose and oxygen, energy failure, ATP depletion and loss of ion exchange function of membrane pumps, terminal depolarization and glutamate-mediated calcium excitotoxicity, calcium-dependent enzyme activation, generation of free radicals, and ultimately degradation of cellular molecules. Both cytotoxic edema (from above) and vasogenic edema (later on from blood-brain barrier disruption) occur in malignant stroke. Identifying individual genetically determined factors of cell death and inflammation could serve as molecular markers of malignant stroke risk in a given patient.

Macroscopic pathology
Within the macroscopic region of infarct, there are well-described zones of decreasing cerebral blood flow and increasing impairment of function[8] (**Fig. 1**). This concept of ischemic penumbra and potentially salvageable brain tissue is central to strategic implementation of therapies including DC. Animal studies have convincingly demonstrated improvement in cortical perfusion, reduction in infarct size, and clinical function following experimental middle cerebral artery (MCA) occlusion.[9] Progressive swelling of infarct tissue leads to transtentorial herniation in a craniocaudal direction and midline shift with subfalcine herniation.[10] Continued swelling can recruit additional arterial territories (posterior and anterior cerebral arteries, respectively) resulting in multiterritory infarction and worsened outcome.

Predictors of Progression

Time since stroke
Cerebral edema progresses during the first 24 to 48 hours after the onset of ischemic stroke and can result in herniation after Day 2[3] (although herniation can occur earlier than this in some cases).

Table 1
Existing evidence on decompressive craniectomy

Trial	Year	Age (y)	No. of Patients (n)	Time to Surgery from Onset of Stroke (h)	Medical Arm Mortality (%)	Medical Arm mRS >4 (%)	Surgical Arm Mortality (%)	Surgical Arm mRS >4 (%)
Destiny-I	2007	18–60	32	12–36	53	73	17.6	53
Decimal	2007	18–55	38	<24	77.8	23	25	50
Hamlet	2009	18–60	64	<96	59	15	22	53
Pooled Analysis	2007	18–60	32	<48	71	7	22	35
Destiny-II	2011	>61	49	<48	70	28	33	60
HeADDFIRST	2014	18–75	26	<96	40	60	21	72

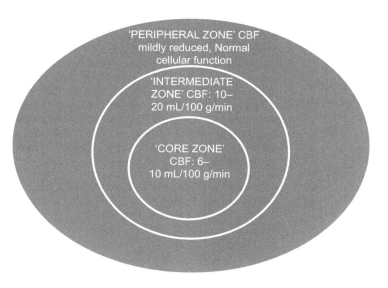

Fig. 1. Zones of cerebral blood flow (CBF).

National Institutes of Health stroke scale

A high initial stroke score, especially involving a score more than 1 on item 1a of the National Institutes of Health stroke scale,[2] has been shown to correlate with an increased risk of progression to malignant edema. Patients with National Institutes of Health stroke scale score of 18 or more on admission are at increased risk of developing malignant cerebral edema.[11]

Computed tomography

A large hypodensity occupying more than two-thirds of the MCA territory is an important predictor of malignant progression.[11] Additional features portending progression include appearance of edema within 6 hours, basal ganglia involvement, dense MCA sign, and midline shift more than 5 mm in the first 2 days.[12–14] The risk of malignant course is estimated by ASPECTS (Alberta Stroke Program Early CT score), where 7 was the cutoff score to determine progression to malignant infarction with 50% sensitivity and 86% specificity.[15] On computed tomography (CT) perfusion maps the early involvement of more than two-thirds of the MCA territory predicted malignant course with 92% sensitivity and 94% specificity.[16]

MRI

An MRI-measured infarct volume of greater than 145 mL on diffusion-weighted imaging done within 14 hours of stroke onset was predictive of clinical deterioration in a study reported by Oppenheim and colleagues.[17]

The risk for malignant stroke progression is likely linked to the quality of the collateral circulation.[17]

Mathematical prediction models incorporating quality of collateral circulation, infarct size, and cellular ischemia response[18–21] have the potential to guide timely institution of early DC.

Best Medical Management

Medical management of patients with malignant MCA infarction specifically is not well defined and follows general management of raised ICP. Most authors have recommended osmotherapy with mannitol or hypertonic saline, head end elevation to 30°, short-term hyperventilation, blood pressure control, maintenance of normal blood glucose, body temperature, and intravascular volume to reduce ICP. Despite best medical management, patients continue to deteriorate and hence it should be considered as a bridge to more definitive therapy, which is surgical decompression consisting of hemicraniectomy. ICP monitoring may help guide management of intracranial hypertension in patients who are not surgical candidates.[22]

Data on Decompressive Craniectomy Before Randomized Controlled Trials

Gupta and colleagues[23] performed a systematic review of 15 studies consisting of a total of 138 patients. The overall mortality in this cohort was 24%, which compared favorably with published reports suggesting mortality of 78% in this patient population. Additionally, 42% of the patients had a good outcome, defined as patients who were independent (7%) or who had mild to moderate disability (35%).

Data from Randomized Controlled Trials on Hemicraniectomy for Malignant Ischemic Stroke

Table 1 is a compilation of the landmark randomized controlled trials (RCTs) comparing DC plus medical management with medical management alone in malignant stroke involving the MCA territory.

Study design

The study design of all six multicenter prospective RCTs was similar with some notable differences.[24–29] Patients were randomized to surgical treatment versus medical management. The trials included patients of less than or equal to 60 years of age except HeADDFIRST (18–75 years). The DESTINY II trial was focused on patients older than 60 years. The primary outcome was defined by the MRS (modified rankin scale) score, which was dichotomized between favorable outcome (0–3) and unfavorable outcome (4–6) in the DECIMAL, DESTINY, and HAMLET trials. In the pooled analysis of 2007 (included patients from the three European RCTs [DECIMAL, DESTINY I, and HAMLET] to reliably predict the effects of surgery with respect to timing [<48 hours] and functional outcome in patients with ischemic stroke[27]) and DESTINY II trial, MRS was dichotomized between 0 and 4 (good outcome) and 5 and 6 (poor outcome). The HeADDFIRST trial reported primary outcome as case fatality at 21 days after treatment.

Surgical technique (craniectomy-duraplasty) was largely similar in all trials. However, the time interval allowed between symptom onset and surgery differed. DC was performed within 24 hours of stroke onset in DECIMAL, 96 hours in HAMLET and HeADDFIRST, 48 hours in DESTINY II, and between 12 and 36 hours in DESTINY I. Another important difference was in imaging selection criteria. DESTINY I and II required infarct size greater than two-thirds of MCA territory (including basal ganglia) on CT, infarct volume greater than 145 cm^3 on diffusion-weighted MRI in DECIMAL, MCA infarct size of at least two-thirds in HAMLET, and greater than 50% of the MCA territory in HeADDFIRST.

Results of the randomized controlled trials

Effects on mortality (MRS 6) All the trials (except HeADDFIRST) showed statistically significant reduction in mortality in surgical patients (**Fig. 2**). DECIMAL and HAMLET showed a statistically significant absolute risk reduction (ARR) of 53% at 6 months (P<.001) and 37% at 1 year (P<.002), respectively. DESTINY I reported 12% mortality in the surgical arm versus 53% in medical arm at 30 days (P = .002). In the pooled analysis, ARR in the surgical arm was found to be 51% (95% confidence interval, 34–69) at 12 months. DESTINY II showed 43% and 76% mortality in the surgical and medical arm, respectively, at 12 months (P<.01).

Effects on moderately severe disability (MRS 4) The pooled analysis and the DESTINY II trial included MRS 4 in the good outcome category with the aim of demonstrating reduced mortality without an increase in severely disabled survivors (MRS 5). A major difference between MRS 4 and 5 is that the latter are completely dependent (including permanent vegetative state). Ultimately

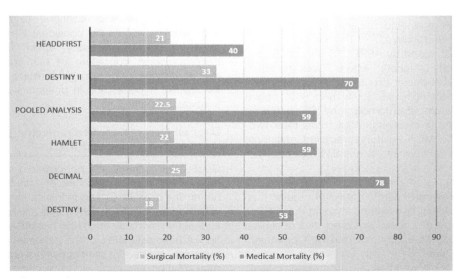

Fig. 2. Mortality rates in percentages.

the pooled analysis results showed greater number of patients in MRS 0 to 4 in the surgical group (76%) versus medical (24%) at 1 year. This means that patients treated with DC have a statistically higher chance of having a good outcome with survival than medically treated survivors. The DESTINY II trial showed similar results (surgical decompression 38% vs medical 18%; $P = .04$). The effect, however, was not as large as in the trials involving younger (<60 years) patients.

Effects on severe disability (MRS 5) DECIMAL, DESTINY, and HAMLET I showed a statistically significant reduction in patients with MRS 5 (severely disabled, bedridden, incontinent, and requiring constant nursing care and attention). In fact, the results of the DECIMAL trial reported no patients with MRS score of 5 at 1 year postsurgery ($P<.0001$). The pooled analysis showed 41.9% (95% confidence interval, 25%–58.6%) ARR for bad outcome with surgery. The DESTINY II trial, however, had 28% patients in MRS 5 after surgery versus 13% after medical management. Although the result was caused by high mortality with medical treatment, it does indicate that DC can result in a significant number of severely disabled survivors in an elderly population (age >60). Further study is needed to determine the utility of DC in this age group. It is possible that further advances in medical therapy, rehabilitation, robotics, and brain computer interfaces will result in better outcomes. At our institution we consider craniectomy in select patients after careful discussion with the patients' surrogates.

Effect on MRS 0 to 3 (good outcome) The pooled analysis showed a statistically significant increase in number of patients in MRS 0 to 3 after surgical decompression versus best medical therapy for patients younger than age 60. These data are compelling and should be communicated in a meaningful way to surrogates of patients who have malignant MCA infraction.

Effect of timing of surgery on outcome HAMLET afforded an opportunity to study the effect of timing on outcomes. Subgroup analyses indicated a far greater benefit of DC in patients operated within 48 hours in reducing the risk of severe disability or death (MRS 5/6; ARR 48%) versus those treated after 48 hours (ARR 27%). The pooled analysis confirmed this, with an ARR for MRS 5/6 of nearly 50% for patients operated within 24 hours. Recent guidelines recommend (class I, level B) performing hemicraniectomy within 48 hours in patients younger than 60 years of age.[2] At our institution we generally favor early

craniectomy for patients who show evidence for malignant MCA infarction based on these data.

Dominant hemisphere involvement
In a subgroup analysis of patients with dominant versus nondominant hemispheric stroke (in the DECIMAL trial), there was no statistically significant difference reported with respect to the primary functional outcomes. Several retrospective studies have reported significant improvement of aphasic symptoms after infarction of speech-dominant hemisphere treated by DC.[30] There are no convincing long-term data in the literature that justify a hemisphere laterality bias in decision-making.

Additional evidence
A critically appraised topic was commissioned in 2011 by Starling and colleagues[31] through development of a clinical scenario, structured clinical questions, search strategy and selection of an article, critical appraisal, evidence summary, clinical bottom lines, and expert commentary from vascular neurologists and a vascular neurosurgeon. They included data on malignant stroke from multicenter randomized trials and an updated meta-analysis. The study concluded that early surgical decompression (within 48 hours of stroke onset) reduces the risks of death and poor clinical outcome at 1 year in patients with large territory cerebral infarction.

Limitations of the randomized controlled trials
There are several limitations associated with these studies. The overall number of patients with good functional outcomes (MRS 0–3) was not statistically significant in the surgical arm (DECIMAL, DESTINY I, and HAMLET). The profile of surgical patients was probably not "real world." For example, the DECIMAL trial excluded patients who were unable to undergo MRI or those who had received tissue plasminogen activator. HAMLET excluded patients who received tissue plasminogen activator within 12 hours of randomization. Patients had to have good baseline functional status as calculated by MRS. Best medical management varied between and within trials. Importantly average time from stroke onset to randomization varied from 24 to 96 hours. None of the investigators grading MRS outcome in DESTINY I and HAMLET were blinded. An overarching limitation is the reliance on MRS to grade outcomes. It is imperative to understand that MRS lends disproportionate importance to gait while neglecting other parameters, such as personal satisfaction, sense of fulfillment, caregiver satisfaction, cognitive function, symptoms of depression, and so forth. For instance, someone in a

wheelchair could be highly productive on a personal and professional level. The significance of cultural differences in addition to the previously mentioned points, in individual cases, should also be recognized.[32–34]

Surgical Technique

We prefer to place the head in rigid three-pin fixation. A large reverse question mark flap is turned to allow access to a large part of the hemicranium. A large craniectomy is performed involving the frontotemporoparietal region without injury to the venous sinuses. Avoiding the frontal air sinus is also preferred to avoid risks of infection and cerebrospinal fluid leak. It is critical to take the inferior bone cut as low as possible to the floor of the middle fossa and ronguer/drill additional bone to accomplish this. A typical craniectomy flap measures at least 15 cm anteroposteriorly and 10 to 12 cm craniocaudal. The dura is opened in a C-shaped or stellate manner. When the anterior temporal lobe is infarcted and tentorial herniation is present or impending, it is our preference to perform an anterior temporal lobectomy with resection of the uncus and visualization of the tentorial edge, third nerve, and midbrain. This reduces brainstem compression in cases of refractory postoperative swelling and likely results in less need to return to the operating room. A lax duraplasty is performed with autologous pericranial graft. The closure must be capacious; one must be able to pick up and freely slide the lax dural sac. Meticulous intradural and epidural hemostasis is achieved. Muscle is reapproximated loosely or not at all. Scalp is closed in layers (drains are optional but often preferred). A parenchymal or subdural ICP monitor is optional. The bone flap is typically discarded because we prefer delayed cranioplasty with a custom implant. Alternately one could store the bone flap in the abdominal wall or cryopreserve it. Postoperatively, we transfer patients to the neurosurgical intensive care unit without extubation.

Postoperative Management

Standard intensive care unit management of increased ICP is carried out. Early extubation without gagging is attempted. Early enteral nutrition is initiated by postoperative Day 1. Subcutaneous heparin is initiated as chemical deep venous thrombosis prophylaxis after 24 hours unless contraindications exist. We have a low threshold for performing early tracheostomy and/or endoscopic percutaneous gastrostomy. With stable postoperative CT, aspirin is initiated after 24 hours. Aggressive physical therapy, speech therapy, and rehabilitation are an integral part of postoperative management.

Complications of Decompressive Craniectomy

Hygroma or subdural fluid collection is the most frequently encountered complication,[25] occurring in 50% to 58% of patients in a study reported by Aarabi and colleagues[35] (most are clinically insignificant). Hydrocephalus is seen as a delayed complication in 7% to 12% of the patients[35,36] and may require shunt placement (our own experience suggests a lower risk than what has been published). Infection is reported between 2% and 7% (our experience suggests this may be closer to 1% and is minimized by avoidance of frontal sinus violation and using pericranium instead of artificial dural substitutes).[35,37] Sinking flap syndrome (syndrome of the trephined) occurs in some patients but is ameliorated by cranioplasty. Overall it is our impression that the complication rate from this procedure is acceptably low and should not be the reason to withhold this life saving procedure for patients who could benefit.

Decompressive Craniectomy for Malignant Middle Cerebral Artery Stroke: A Case Illustration

A 61-year-old man presented with acute right hemiplegia caused by embolic occlusion of right M1 following recent aortic root surgery. CT revealed large right MCA territory infarct (>2/3) (**Fig. 3**). Because of large infarct size and high mortality with medical management, a decision to proceed with DC was made after discussion with family (**Fig. 4**). He demonstrated excellent recovery following DC. Cranioplasty with custom implant was performed (**Fig. 5**). His 5-month MRS was 3. He and his family were happy that every effort was made to save his life in the acute setting including performance of DC.

ISCHEMIC POSTERIOR FOSSA STROKE (INFRATENTORIAL)

Space-occupying edema is reported to occur in 17% to 54% of patients with cerebellar infarction.[38] Life-threatening brainstem compression may develop rapidly in the limited confines of the posterior fossa. Surgical options vary from ventriculostomy (external ventricular drain [EVD]) placement alone (no longer recommended as a stand-alone treatment in most cases), craniectomy with duraplasty, or both. In such patients ventriculostomy should always be accompanied or followed by craniectomy (class I, level C) for the treatment of obstructive hydrocephalus after a cerebellar

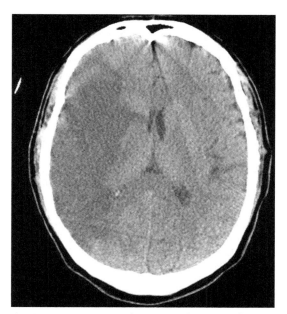

Fig. 3. Preoperative CT showing right MCA infarct.

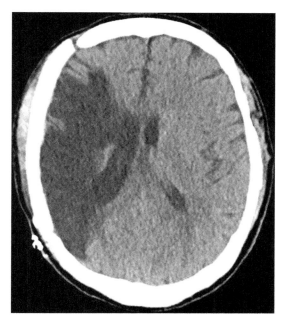

Fig. 5. CT postcranioplasty.

infarct.[2] No RCTs comparing the efficacy of various surgical approaches, timing of surgery, or data on long-term functional outcomes have been published. However, resection of ischemic/necrotic tissue (strokectomy) is often added to craniectomy and have led to class I, level B recommendation for performing suboccipital craniectomy in neurologically deteriorating patients despite best medical management.[2]

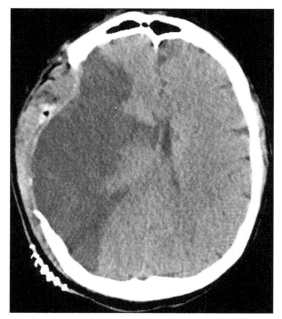

Fig. 4. Postoperative CT.

Existing Evidence

Most data in the literature regarding the efficacy of craniectomy in space-occupying cerebellar infarcts is retrospective and are mostly single center experiences. Juttler and colleagues[38] performed a retrospective study of 56 consecutive patients with cerebellar infarction and studied long-term outcome (minimum 3 years) in surgically treated patients (EVD, suboccipital decompression, or both). The study reported an overall 39% mortality. Of the survivors, 52% had favorable functional outcome (MRS 0–3) at 3-year follow-up. There were no significant differences in mortality or functional outcome observed between surgical treatment groups.[38] Pfefferkorn and colleagues[39] studied 57 patients who underwent surgery, at a wide range of follow-up (1–11 years). A total of 40% died at long-term follow-up. More than half of survivors had good outcome. Presence of brainstem infarction was associated with poor outcome. Tsitsopoulos and colleagues[40] looked into 32 patients treated uniformly with EVD, craniectomy, and "strokectomy." Presence of Glasgow Coma Score less than or equal to 13 and signs of posterior fossa mass effect were criteria for surgery. Six-month mortality was 12.5%. At long-term follow-up (median, 67.5 months), nearly 70% were alive and of them, nearly 77% had good outcome (MRS 0–2). More than half of those older than 70 years of age had a good outcome. One-third of patients who were comatose before surgery had a good outcome. A small retrospective study reported good long-term outcomes in surgical patients (6 of total 10) with bilateral cerebellar infarcts but without brainstem infarcts.[41] These studies are unfortunately plagued by inevitable bias (depending on severity of mass effect, clinical profile, and treating team) in a retrospectively analyzed patient population. Many of these studies did not include MRI before surgery.

One of the few prospective studies (nonrandomized) was conducted by Jauss and colleagues[42] (German-Austrian cerebellar infarction study) and included 84 patients with cerebellar stroke. The study concluded that surgery provided benefit only in comatose patients (and not in awake/drowsy or somnolent/drowsy regardless of infarct size). Level of consciousness was the strongest predictor of outcome. A total of 76% of patients had a good outcome (MRS 0–2) in the surgical group.

Most authors agree that waiting to perform surgery until a patient becomes comatose is not standard practice. It seems prudent to proceed with surgical decompression with a tight posterior fossa, before significant decline in sensorium is clinically evident to maximize recovery of neurologic function. Accepted criteria for a tight posterior fossa include fourth ventricle compression, hydrocephalus, and effacement of quadrigeminal cistern.[42]

Surgical Technique

Surgery begins with frontal ventriculostomy (if not already in place) and then turning the patient prone with three-pin head fixation. It is our preference to avoid cerebrospinal fluid drainage until the craniectomy is performed to avoid the risks of upward herniation. A standard midline or lateral suboccipital incision from level of inion to C2 is made and suboccipital bone, posterior C1 arch, and C2 upper lamina is exposed. A wide craniectomy, extending across the midline if necessary, is made along with C1 arch resection, followed by dural opening. Herniating infarcted tissue is resected and hemostasis achieved. A wide duraplasty is performed with pericranium and/or other dural substitute and closure is performed in layers. Postoperative intensive care unit management proceeds in standard fashion. If attempts to wean the EVD are unsuccessful, a shunt or in some instances an endoscopic third ventriculostomy is necessary.

Decompressive Craniectomy for Posterior Fossa Ischemic Stroke: A Case Illustration

A 52-year-old man presented with acute right cerebellar infarct caused by posterior inferior cerebellar–vertebral artery occlusion. Rapid cerebellar swelling occurred during the next 24 hours (**Fig. 6**) and posterior fossa DC (including strokectomy) with EVD placement was performed (**Fig. 7**). He improved excellently and was weaned from EVD. His long-term (5 year) follow-up MRS was 1.

HEMORRHAGIC STROKE
Overview of Intracerebral Hemorrhage

Hemorrhagic stroke accounts for approximately 10% to 20% of all strokes.[43] The term most often connotes spontaneous ICH (SICH) and excludes hemorrhage from structural causes, such as aneurysm, arteriovenous malformation, and tumor. However, the applicability of DC to ICH from all etiologies is similar. We prefer the term SICH rather than hemorrhagic stroke. Hypertension is the most common cause of SICH.

Pathophysiology of Spontaneous Intracerebral Hemorrhage

Neurologic adverse effects from ICH result from mass effect of the hematoma and from a cascade of cellular events. The latter are triggered from heme degradation products and plasma components from extravasated blood. This incites proinflammatory cytokine-mediated reactions via macrophages, white cells, mast cells, and microglia. Subsequent damage occurs via free radical–mediated cellular degradation, apoptosis, autophagy, and matrix metalloproteinase–mediated disruption of blood-brain barrier.[44] Hematoma expansion in the early period after hemorrhage is a major cause of neurologic morbidity and mortality.[45] In addition, perihematoma edema seen on

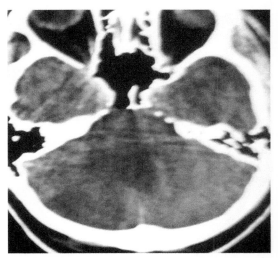

Fig. 6. Preoperative CT showing right cerebellar infarct.

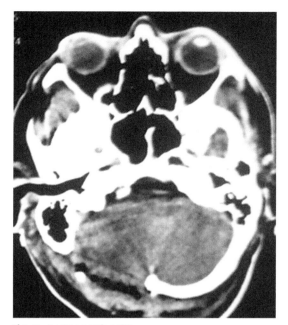

Fig. 7. Postoperative CT.

neuroimaging grows rapidly in the first 48 hours after the onset of hemorrhagic stroke.[17] Both expansion of hematoma and perihematoma edema have the potential to cause significant, even catastrophic, increases in ICP and fatal herniation.

Decompressive Craniectomy for Supratentorial Intracerebral Hemorrhage

DC is a valuable tool for controlling ICP in large SICH. The latest American Heart Association/American Stroke Association guidelines on the management of SICH published in 2015 suggest a favorable outcome with "Decompressive craniectomy (with or without hematoma evacuation) performed in patients with supratentorial ICH with midline shift or increased ICP refractory to medical treatment" (class IIb, level C).[46] This recommendation was based on several studies. Fung and colleagues[47] reported a retrospective study of DC without hematoma evacuation. This study matched 12 patients with supratentorial ICH to control subjects and found a 25% mortality rate (3 of 12) compared with the control group, which had 53% mortality rate (8 of 15). Hayes and colleagues[48] published a retrospective study on DC in 2013. This study included surgical evacuation of the hematoma in addition to DC and found that patients in the surgical group had a strong trend toward good neurologic outcome (MRS <3). A systematic review on DC in addition to hematoma evacuation has shown favorable outcomes in patients with ICH.[49] There have been

some concerns raised about DC worsening hematoma expansion but these have mostly been retrospective observations in the typical time frame wherein natural hematoma expansion occurs.[46]

Decompressive Craniectomy for Hemorrhagic Stroke: A Case Illustration

A 52-year-old hypertensive woman presented with lethargy and acute right hemiparesis and aphasia. CT revealed a large 4 × 4.2 × 6 cm ICH in the dominant (left) posterior frontal region with 6-mm midline shift, mass effect, and hemispheric edema (**Fig. 8**). Urgent CT and catheter angiogram were negative. Left DC and clot evacuation was performed. Postoperatively she rapidly improved in speech and hemiparesis, and was discharged to rehabilitation (**Fig. 9**). Her 3-month MRS was 2 and successful cranioplasty was performed.

Decompressive Craniectomy for Posterior Fossa Hemorrhage

Surgery for cerebellar hematoma is probably least controversial across neurovascular teams around the world. Hematoma evacuation is standard practice and the extent of brain relaxation following clot evacuation is usually more dramatic than during surgery for ischemic stroke. DC therefore becomes part of the surgery to allow room for potential postoperative swelling. The American Heart Association/American Stroke Association guidelines provide level 1, class B recommendations for direct surgical evacuation of cerebellar ICH greater than 3 cm.[46] Location of hematoma may be more influential than size per se; close proximity and pressure on the brainstem lowers the threshold for surgery.

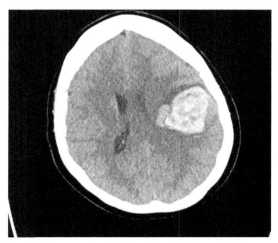

Fig. 8. Preoperative CT showing left frontal ICH.

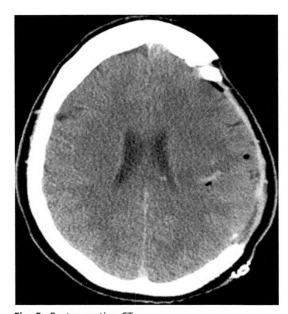

Fig. 9. Postoperative CT.

STATE OF CURRENT KNOWLEDGE AND FUTURE TRIAL AREAS

Malignant MCA infarction has a poor outcome with lone medical management and high mortality rates of 50% to 80%. DC performed within 48 hours in patients with malignant edema younger than 60 years has strong evidence for improving survival and functional outcome (class I, level B).[2] The guidelines acknowledge that the optimal trigger for DC is unknown and suggest decline in consciousness despite maximal medical therapy to serve thus (class IIa, level A).[2] However the evidence is clear enough to consider DC early on in the clinical course instead of waiting for clinical deterioration, to optimize neurologic function. The ideal time window for selection remains elusive, ensuring timely DC on patients who will deteriorate versus avoiding unnecessary surgery in patients whose edema will not progress and may respond to medical therapy alone. Larger well-designed randomized trials, risk stratification algorithms, and mathematical models are worthy future areas for investigation. DC for SICH has weaker evidence but this should not deter the neurovascular team from performing DC as an ICP control tool (with/without ICH evacuation) on salvageable patients with a large clot and hemispheric edema. The decision to operate in patients older than 60 years of age with ischemic hemispheric stroke should be made on an individualized basis. A strategic and clear discussion with family is as critical as the science behind the surgery.

ACKNOWLEDGMENTS

The authors thank Matthew E. Welz, MS, Mayo Clinic, Phoenix, AZ for assistance with the preparation of this article.

REFERENCES

1. Simard JM, Sahuquillo J, Sheth KN, et al. Managing malignant cerebral infarction. Curr Treat Options Neurol 2011;13(2):217–29.
2. Wijdicks EF, Sheth KN, Carter BS, et al. Recommendations for the management of cerebral and cerebellar infarction with swelling: a statement for healthcare professionals from the American Heart Association/American Stroke Association. Stroke 2014;45(4):1222–38.
3. Qureshi AI, Suarez JI, Yahia AM, et al. Timing of neurologic deterioration in massive middle cerebral artery infarction: a multicenter review. Crit Care Med 2003;31(1):272–7.
4. Haring HP, Dilitz E, Pallua A, et al. Attenuated corticomedullary contrast: an early cerebral computed tomography sign indicating malignant middle cerebral artery infarction. A case-control study. Stroke 1999;30(5):1076–82.
5. Minnerup J, Wersching H, Ringelstein EB, et al. Prediction of malignant middle cerebral artery infarction using computed tomography-based intracranial volume reserve measurements. Stroke 2011;42(12):3403–9.
6. Hacke W, Schwab S, Horn M, et al. 'Malignant' middle cerebral artery territory infarction: clinical course and prognostic signs. Arch Neurol 1996;53(4):309–15.
7. Broughton BR, Reutens DC, Sobey CG. Apoptotic mechanisms after cerebral ischemia. Stroke 2009;40(5):e331–9.
8. Symon L, Pasztor E, Branston N. The distribution and density of reduced cerebral blood flow following acute middle cerebral artery occlusion: an experimental study by the technique of hydrogen clearance in baboons. Stroke 1974;5(3):355–64.
9. Doerfler A, Engelhorn T, Heiland S, et al. Perfusion- and diffusion-weighted magnetic resonance imaging for monitoring decompressive craniectomy in animals with experimental hemispheric stroke. J Neurosurg 2002;96(5):933–40.
10. Youmans JR. Neurological surgery; a comprehensive reference guide to the diagnosis and management of neurosurgical problems. Philadelphia: Saunders; 1973.
11. Krieger DW, Demchuk AM, Kasner SE, et al. Early clinical and radiological predictors of fatal brain swelling in ischemic stroke. Stroke 1999;30(2):287–92.
12. Kucinski T, Koch C, Grzyska U, et al. The predictive value of early CT and angiography for fatal

hemispheric swelling in acute stroke. AJNR Am J Neuroradiol 1998;19(5):839–46.

13. Manno EM, Nichols DA, Fulgham JR, et al. Computed tomographic determinants of neurologic deterioration in patients with large middle cerebral artery infarctions. Mayo Clin Proc 2003; 78(2):156–60.

14. Pullicino PM, Alexandrov AV, Shelton JA, et al. Mass effect and death from severe acute stroke. Neurology 1997;49(4):1090–5.

15. MacCallum C, Churilov L, Mitchell P, et al. Low Alberta Stroke Program Early CT score (ASPECTS) associated with malignant middle cerebral artery infarction. Cerebrovasc Dis 2014;38(1):39–45.

16. Ryoo JW, Na DG, Kim SS, et al. Malignant middle cerebral artery infarction in hyperacute ischemic stroke: evaluation with multiphasic perfusion computed tomography maps. J Comput Assist Tomogr 2004;28(1):55–62.

17. Oppenheim C, Samson Y, Manai R, et al. Prediction of malignant middle cerebral artery infarction by diffusion-weighted imaging. Stroke 2000;31(9): 2175–81.

18. Tegos TJ, Kalodiki E, Daskalopoulou SS, et al. Stroke: epidemiology, clinical picture, and risk factors: part I of III. Angiology 2000;51(10):793–808.

19. Rowley HA. The four Ps of acute stroke imaging: parenchyma, pipes, perfusion, and penumbra. AJNR Am J Neuroradiol 2001;22(4):599–601.

20. Thanvi B, Treadwell S, Robinson T. Early neurological deterioration in acute ischaemic stroke: predictors, mechanisms and management. Postgrad Med J 2008;84(994):412–7.

21. Gretarsdottir S, Thorleifsson G, Reynisdottir ST, et al. The gene encoding phosphodiesterase 4D confers risk of ischemic stroke. Nat Genet 2003;35(2):131–8.

22. El Ahmadieh TY, Adel JG, El Tecle NE, et al. Surgical treatment of elevated intracranial pressure: decompressive craniectomy and intracranial pressure monitoring. Neurosurg Clin N Am 2013;24(3):375–91.

23. Gupta R, Connolly ES, Mayer S, et al. Hemicraniectomy for massive middle cerebral artery territory infarction a systematic review. Stroke 2004;35(2): 539–43.

24. Vahedi K, Vicaut E, Mateo J, et al. Sequential-design, multicenter, randomized, controlled trial of early decompressive craniectomy in malignant middle cerebral artery infarction (DECIMAL Trial). Stroke 2007;38(9):2506–17.

25. Juttler E, Schwab S, Schmiedek P, et al. Decompressive surgery for the treatment of malignant infarction of the middle cerebral artery (DESTINY): a randomized, controlled trial. Stroke 2007;38(9):2518–25.

26. Hofmeijer J, Kappelle LJ, Algra A, et al. Surgical decompression for space-occupying cerebral infarction (the Hemicraniectomy After Middle Cerebral Artery infarction with Life-threatening Edema Trial [HAMLET]): a multicentre, open, randomised trial. Lancet Neurol 2009;8(4):326–33.

27. Vahedi K, Hofmeijer J, Juettler E, et al. Early decompressive surgery in malignant infarction of the middle cerebral artery: a pooled analysis of three randomised controlled trials. Lancet Neurol 2007; 6(3):215–22.

28. Juttler E, Unterberg A, Woitzik J, et al. Hemicraniectomy in older patients with extensive middle-cerebral-artery stroke. N Engl J Med 2014;370(12): 1091–100.

29. Frank JI, Schumm LP, Wroblewski K, et al. Hemicraniectomy and durotomy upon deterioration from infarction-related swelling trial: randomized pilot clinical trial. Stroke 2014;45(3):781–7.

30. Sundseth J, Sundseth A, Thommessen B, et al. Long-term outcome and quality of life after craniectomy in speech-dominant swollen middle cerebral artery infarction. Neurocrit Care 2015; 22(1):6–14.

31. Starling AJ, Wellik KE, Snyder CRH, et al. Surgical decompression improves mortality and morbidity after large territory acute cerebral infarction: a critically appraised topic. Neurologist 2011; 17(1):63–6.

32. Rahme R, Zuccarello M, Kleindorfer D, et al. Decompressive hemicraniectomy for malignant middle cerebral artery territory infarction: is life worth living? Clinical article. J Neurosurg 2012;117(4):749–54.

33. Ragoschke-Schumm A, Junk C, Lesmeister M, et al. Retrospective consent to hemicraniectomy after malignant stroke among the elderly, despite impaired functional outcome. Cerebrovasc Dis 2015;40(5–6): 286–92.

34. Honeybul S, Ho KM, Blacker DW. ORACLE Stroke Study: opinion regarding acceptable outcome following decompressive hemicraniectomy for ischemic stroke. Neurosurgery 2016;79(2):231–6.

35. Aarabi B, Chesler D, Maulucci C, et al. Dynamics of subdural hygroma following decompressive craniectomy: a comparative study. Neurosurg Focus 2009;26(6):E8.

36. Yang XF, Wen L, Shen F, et al. Surgical complications secondary to decompressive craniectomy in patients with a head injury: a series of 108 consecutive cases. Acta Neurochir (Wien) 2008;150(12): 1241–7 [discussion: 1248].

37. Aarabi B, Hesdorffer DC, Ahn ES, et al. Outcome following decompressive craniectomy for malignant swelling due to severe head injury. J Neurosurg 2006;104(4):469–79.

38. Juttler E, Schweickert S, Ringleb PA, et al. Long-term outcome after surgical treatment for space-occupying cerebellar infarction: experience in 56 patients. Stroke 2009;40(9):3060–6.

39. Pfefferkorn T, Eppinger U, Linn J, et al. Long-term outcome after suboccipital decompressive

craniectomy for malignant cerebellar infarction. Stroke 2009;40(9):3045–50.

40. Tsitsopoulos PP, Tobieson L, Enblad P, et al. Surgical treatment of patients with unilateral cerebellar infarcts: clinical outcome and prognostic factors. Acta Neurochir 2011;153(10):2075–83.

41. Tsitsopoulos P, Tobieson L, Enblad P, et al. Clinical outcome following surgical treatment for bilateral cerebellar infarction. Acta Neurol Scand 2011; 123(5):345–51.

42. Jauss M, Krieger D, Hornig C, et al. Surgical and medical management of patients with massive cerebellar infarctions: results of the German-Austrian Cerebellar Infarction Study. J Neurol 1999;246(4): 257–64.

43. Liu F, Yuan R, Benashski SE, et al. Changes in experimental stroke outcome across the life span. J Cereb Blood Flow Metab 2009;29(4):792–802.

44. Grotta JC, Albers GW, Broderick JP, et al. Stroke: pathophysiology, diagnosis, and management. Elsevier Health Sciences; 2016.

45. Delcourt C, Huang Y, Arima H, et al. Hematoma growth and outcomes in intracerebral hemorrhage. The INTERACT1 study. Neurology 2012;79(4):314–9.

46. Hemphill JC 3rd, Greenberg SM, Anderson CS, et al. Guidelines for the management of spontaneous intracerebral hemorrhage: a guideline for healthcare professionals from the American Heart Association/American Stroke Association. Stroke 2015;46(7):2032–60.

47. Fung C, Murek M, Z'Graggen WJ, et al. Decompressive hemicraniectomy in patients with supratentorial intracerebral hemorrhage. Stroke 2012;43(12): 3207–11.

48. Hayes SB, Benveniste RJ, Morcos JJ, et al. Retrospective comparison of craniotomy and decompressive craniectomy for surgical evacuation of nontraumatic, supratentorial intracerebral hemorrhage. Neurosurg Focus 2013;34(5):E3.

49. Takeuchi S, Wada K, Nagatani K, et al. Decompressive hemicraniectomy for spontaneous intracerebral hemorrhage. Neurosurg Focus 2013;34(5):E5.

Direct Versus Indirect Bypass for Moyamoya Disease

Jonathan J. Liu, MD[a], Gary K. Steinberg, MD, PhD[b],*

KEYWORDS

- Direct bypass • EDAS • Indirect bypass • Moyamoya • Omental transposition

KEY POINTS

- Surgical revascularization is the main therapy for moyamoya disease, as it prevents risk of future stroke.
- Surgical options can be divided into indirect, direct, or combined approaches.
- In general, a direct bypass is performed in patients with occlusive disease (occlusion of internal carotid artery [ICA] or middle cerebral artery [MCA]).
- In general, an indirect bypass is reserved for patients with stenosis and not occlusion of the ICA or MCA, and in cases when the donor or recipient arteries are too small.
- Competing flows after a direct bypass may cause stagnation in the existing collateral supply or occasionally accelerate occlusion of an already stenosed native circulation.

INTRODUCTION

In 1957, Takeuchi and Shimizu[1] first described a progressive occlusive vasculopathy that involves the supraclinoid internal carotid arteries and Circle of Willis and results in the formation of arterial collaterals at the skull base. In 1969, Suzuki and Takaku[2] termed this network of collateral formation seen on angiography as "moyamoya," meaning "puff of smoke" in Japanese.

Moyamoya disease is now widely accepted as a disease process that not only affects patients of Asian descent, but is also prevalent in North America and Europe. Familial cases account for approximately 15% of the disease.[3] In 2012, Starke and colleagues[4] analyzed the moyamoya patients admitted to US hospitals from 2002 to 2008 using the National Inpatient Sample. A total of 2280 patients were admitted with a diagnosis of moyamoya disorder, which translated to an incidence of 0.57 per 100,000 persons per year. This was considerably higher than the incidence of 0.086 per 100,000 persons per year in Washington State and California from 1987 to 1998.[5]

In Japan, a recent analysis of patients with moyamoya disease admitted in 2003 yielded an annual rate of 0.54 per 100,000, which was close to the findings of Starke and colleagues[4] in North America. The prevalence of moyamoya disease in Japan nearly doubled with almost a 100% increase from 3900 patients in 1994 to 7700 cases in 2003. It is, however, difficult to determine if this increase in prevalence represents increased

Disclosure Statement: This work was funded in part by Bernard Lacroute, Ronni Lacroute, the William Randolph Hearst Foundation, and Russell and Beth Siegelman (to G.K. Steinberg). We declare no conflict of interest related to this study. Dr G.K. Steinberg is a consultant for Qool Therapeutics, Peter Lazic US, Inc, and NeuroSave.

[a] Department of Neurosurgery, Stanford University School of Medicine, R200, 300 Pasteur Drive, Stanford, CA 94305-5327, USA; [b] Department of Neurosurgery, Stanford University School of Medicine, R281, 300 Pasteur Drive, Stanford, CA 94305-5327, USA
* Corresponding author.
E-mail address: gsteinberg@stanford.edu

awareness and improved diagnostic measures or an actual increase in disease incidence.[6]

The pathophysiology of moyamoya disease remains unclear. Pathologic specimens have shown that the outer diameters of the carotid artery are diminutive with increased intimal thickening.[7] Caspase-3–dependent apoptosis has been implicated as a possible contributor to the pathophysiology of moyamoya disease.[8] Fibrin deposition along with the elastic laminae abnormalities and microaneurysm formation within the dilated moyamoya vessels may contribute to intracranial hemorrhage in these patients. Conversely, stenosed moyamoya vessels can lead to thrombosis and subsequent brain ischemia.[9,10] Children in Asian populations tend to present with brain ischemia due to inadequate moyamoya collateral formation and nearly 50% of adults present with intracerebral hemorrhage due to the fragility of the collateral vessels that have formed over time.[11,12] Outside of Asia, moyamoya disease may have different phenotypical considerations.[13–15] In the North American cohort, only 14.6% of adults and 2.1% of children presented with hemorrhage,[16] and of 902 patients at Stanford with moyamoya disease, 16% of adults and 6% of pediatric patients presented with hemorrhage.

PATIENT EVALUATION OVERVIEW

At Stanford, all patients obtain an MRI brain, MR perfusion with and without Diamox, 6-vessel angiogram, neuropsychiatric testing, and surgical clearance from the anesthesia team before surgery. In patients with bilateral moyamoya disease, the more symptomatic hemisphere is treated first. The contralateral hemisphere is usually treated 1 week later, assuming the first surgery was uneventful. Initial surgical laterality is dependent on the patient's clinical symptomatology with associated MRI findings of infarcts and/or poor cerebral blood flow augmentation after administration of acetazolamide (Diamox). A more ominous finding after Diamox administration is a steal phenomenon in which a paradoxic decrease in regional blood flow occurs likely related to maximal arterial dilation in some regions at baseline. We believe these patients are at highest risk for future strokes and require strict blood pressure management in the perioperative period. A contraindication to planned surgery is the presence of an acute (DWI +/ADC+ [Diffusion weighted imaging (DWI); apparent diffusion coefficient (ADC)]) or subacute (DWI+/ADC−) infarct, even a very small one.[17]

NONSURGICAL TREATMENT OPTIONS

Nonsurgical medical therapy using aspirin, mannitol, steroids, and vasodilators have been largely unsuccessful.[18] Left untreated, 23.8% to nearly 49.0% of patients have symptomatic progression over 6 years.[19–21] In a 2007 Japanese multicenter survey, outcomes in asymptomatic patients with untreated moyamoya disease showed a 3.2% annual risk for any stroke.[22] A similar study conducted in North America demonstrated an annual ischemic stroke rate of 13.3% and a hemorrhage rate of 1.7%.[23] Other approaches include intravenous infusion of calcium channel blockers, such as nimodipine or verapamil, which have provided symptomatic improvement in patients with moyamoya disease. Their efficacy, however, has not yet been proven.[24]

Endovascular therapy has also been attempted to help reestablish immediate blood flow to the oxygen-deprived brain. Khan and colleagues[25] reviewed the results of angioplasty and stenting on 5 adult patients, all of whom went on to develop repeated ischemic attacks despite treatment (**Fig. 1**). Although cerebral blood flow may have improved in the short term, 70% to 90% in stent stenosis in 4 patients and occlusion in 1 patient on follow-up angiograms proved this method of treatment was not sustainable. All patients went on to receive a revascularization procedure.

SURGICAL TREATMENT OPTIONS

Medical therapy as the sole treatment modality has been largely supplanted by surgical revascularization procedures due to the ongoing risk of cerebral ischemia or hemorrhage.

In general, cerebral revascularization surgery can be divided into 3 categories:

1. Direct revascularization
2. Indirect revascularization using adjacent or distant vascularized tissue
3. Combined techniques (direct plus indirect)

Direct Bypass Technique

Superficial temporal artery to middle cerebral artery (STA-MCA) bypass has been used since 1973 by Kikuchi and Karasawa[26] and remains the procedure of choice when direct revascularization is desired.[27] Direct revascularization has the added benefit of immediately augmenting blood flow to the oxygen-deprived brain by suturing an extracranial artery directly to cortical branches on the brain surface.

At Stanford, we make an attempt to perform direct bypasses on all patients who are symptomatic with occlusion of the internal carotid artery (ICA) or MCA. Because we harvest a generous cuff of vascularized soft tissue surrounding a long

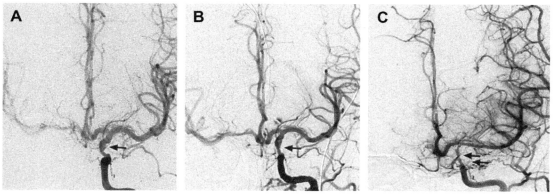

Fig. 1. Failure of endovascular stenting in a patient with moyamoya disease presenting with left hemisphere TIAs. (*A*) Anteroposterior projection of the left ICA demonstrating 70% stenosis of the supraclinoid ICA (*arrow*). (*B*) Residual 30% ICA stenosis after stenting (*arrow*). (*C*) Stent failure 6 months after treatment with worsened 90% ICA stenosis and recurrent TIAs (*arrows*). (*From* Khan N, Dodd R, Marks MP, et al. Failure of primary percutaneous angioplasty and stenting in the prevention of ischemia in Moyamoya angiopathy. Cerebrovasc Dis 2011;31(2):151; with permission.)

segment of scalp artery and then place this in intimate contact with the brain surface in addition to the direct anastomosis, indirect revascularization also occurs over the next 3 to 6 months. All procedures are done under mild hypothermia to target a core temperature of 33°C for neuroprotection. Monitoring of intraoperative electroencephalogram is an important adjunct to surgery, particularly during clamping of the recipient vessel and when confirmation of burst suppression is used before performing the anastomosis.

Both the frontal or parietal branch of the STA can be used for anastomosis and preoperative angiogram aids in choosing the appropriate donor vessel. In general, the parietal branch is used when the vessel diameter is adequate. Too large of a parietal branch is also not desirable, as flow from the donor vessel that is too robust can lead to competing blood flow with the native collateral circulation and promote ischemia, or in rare cases cerebral hyperperfusion. The natural course of the parietal branch also facilitates a craniotomy over the frontotemporal region to better expose M4 vessels emerging from the Sylvian fissure.

The patient is positioned supine with the head turned away from the surgical side and fixated in a Mayfield head holder. Typically, a shoulder roll is placed to prevent excessive neck turning that can result in decreased venous outflow and is particularly important in patients with Down syndrome who may be predisposed to craniocervical instability. The STA branch of interest is then insonated using a handheld Doppler to map the course of the donor vessel (**Fig. 2**). We typically begin mapping the STA above the zygomatic arch. If the parietal branch is chosen, the frontal branch

is preserved should another revascularization procedure be needed in the future.

- Usually a curvilinear incision is planned over the STA. Under high magnification, the initial dissection begins at the proximal STA. The dissection is carried out superficially through the dermis and subcutaneous tissue using Littler scissors. Hemostasis in the dermis can be controlled using low current bipolar electrocautery.

- Small hook retractors are used to facilitate exposure as the dissection is carried toward the convexity. Throughout the dissection, patency of the STA is periodically monitored using the handheld Doppler. Papaverine can be used to prevent STA spasm during dissection. We aim to dissect out approximately 9 cm of STA before creating a vascular cuff that will serve as a means for additional indirect collaterals on the brain surface.

- After the STA has been isolated from the underlying temporalis fascia, self-retaining retractors are placed to prepare for the craniotomy. The temporalis fascia and muscle are then incised in an H-shaped fashion using monopolar electrocautery and carefully lifted off the skull. The assistant surgeon helps protect the STA during muscle dissection and craniotomy to avoid iatrogenic injury to the donor vessel.

- A 6 × 6 cm craniotomy is then created over the frontotemporal region with a burr hole strategically placed at the most inferior aspect to serve as a conduit for STA passage into the intracranial space.

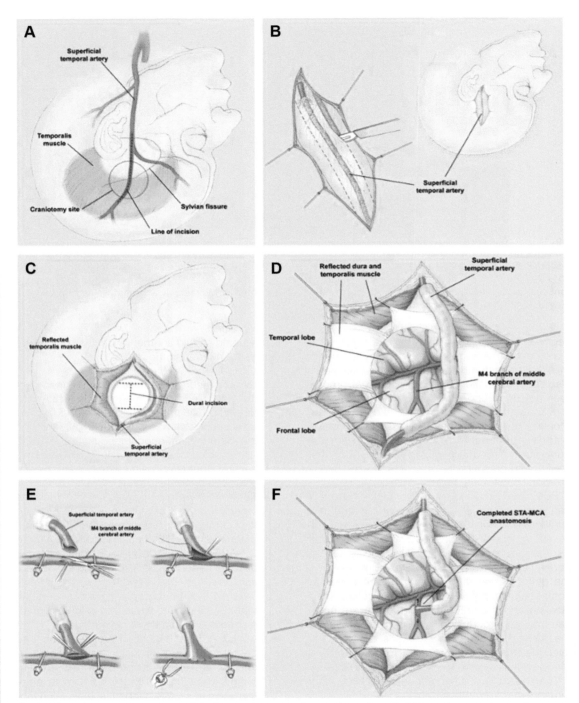

Fig. 2. Direct bypass surgery steps. (A) The STA is mapped out using a handheld Doppler anterior to the zygomatic arch for 8 to 9 cm. (B) The STA and vascular cuff are dissected free under the operating microscope. (C) The temporalis muscle is incised in an H-shaped fashion. A 6 × 6-cm craniotomy is made over the frontotemporal region. (D) The dura is widely opened over the Sylvian fissure. Under high magnification, an M4 recipient artery emerging from the Sylvian fissure is identified. (E) The distal STA is cut at 45° and temporary clips are placed on the recipient artery. An elliptical arteriotomy is made over the M4 branch. An end to side anastomosis is performed using 10 to 0 interrupted suture under high magnification. Once the bypass is completed, temporary clips are removed from the recipient and proximal STA. (F) The STA and vascularized cuff are placed in close apposition to the cortical surface to facilitate delayed collateral formation. (*From* Guzman R, Steinberg GK. Direct bypass techniques for the treatment of pediatric moyamoya disease. Neurosurg Clin N Am 2010;21(3):565–73; with permission.)

- A short segment (~0.5 cm) of the proximal STA just distal to the origin of the frontal branch is prepared by removing all adherent soft tissue to accommodate placement of a temporary clip. Next, 1 cm of the most distal part of the STA is then prepared in a similar fashion using fine micro scissors.
- The dura is then opened in a stellate fashion and tacked up. Under high magnification, the arachnoid is opened to identify an appropriate recipient artery. We aim to find an M4 artery emerging from the Sylvian fissure that is preferentially ≥0.8 mm and also perpendicular to the Sylvian fissure, if possible (**Fig. 3**).
- Once isolated from the underlying cortex, blood flow is measured in the cortical MCA branch and cut STA using an ultrasonic quantitative and directional flow probe (Charbel microflow probe; Transonics Systems, Inc, Ithaca, NY). A high-visibility background is then placed beneath the recipient artery.
- A 45° cut is made at the distal STA and flushed with heparinized saline while the proximal STA is temporarily clipped. Before temporary clipping of the recipient artery, burst suppression is achieved along with a mean arterial pressure of 90 to 100 mm Hg.
- Lazic temporary clips (Peter Lazic GmbH, Tuttlingen, Germany) are then applied on the recipient artery proximal and distal to the planned anastomosis.
- An elliptical arteriotomy is made on the cortical vessel and stained with methylene blue or indigo carmine. An end-to-side microanastomosis is then completed with the use of Monosof suture (10–0) (Covidien, Dublin, Ireland). We prefer an interrupted suture technique, starting with the initial toe stitch followed by a heel stitch. Stitches are placed evenly apart (usually 3 on each side in addition to the 2 end stitches), ensuring not to catch the back wall of the recipient artery with each suture. Once the anastomosis is complete, the temporary clips are first removed from the recipient artery followed by the proximal STA.
- Using the Charbel microflow probe, the quantitative blood flow and its directionality in relation to the Sylvian fissure is measured in the recipient artery both proximal and distal to the anastomosis. A final measurement of the distal STA blood flow after the bypass is also recorded. Finally, the patency of the bypass is confirmed using intraoperative indocyanine green (ICG) video angiography.
- For closure, the dural leaflets are reapproximated loosely, ensuring not to compromise

the parent STA. The bone flap is replaced with the inferior burr hole serving as an unobstructed passageway for the STA to enter the intracranial space. Doppler ultrasound is recommended throughout the closure to make certain no flow-limiting stenosis/occlusion of the STA has occurred during final closure.

Indirect Bypass Techniques

Indirect bypass techniques afford the neurosurgeon alternative methods to revascularize the brain. Indirect procedures rely solely on delayed collateral formation from juxtaposed tissue (eg, intact scalp artery, muscle, pericranium, galea, dura, omentum) on the brain surface over time. Unlike direct bypasses that provide immediate blood flow to a specific vascular territory, indirect methods form collaterals over time and can be tailored to address more than one vascular territory if needed. The procedural and perioperative morbidity associated with patients with moyamoya disease can also be minimized as indirect techniques are typically shorter in duration and less technically demanding.

Techniques have evolved over time, with newer methods building on existing techniques. Indirect techniques vary widely depending on which adjacent tissue is used for synangiosis. These include the following:

- Encephaloduroarteriosynangiosis (EDAS)
- Encephalomyosynangiosis (EMS)
- Encephaloduroarteriomyosynangiosis (EDAMS): a combination of both EDAS and EMS
- Split duro-encephalo-synangiosis (DES)
- Pial synangiosis
- Ribbon EDAMS
- Multiple burr holes (MBH)

Distant omental transposition is an alternative indirect technique when additional blood flow is needed and other direct/indirect measures have been exhausted.

These methods take advantage of the inherent tendency of patients with moyamoya disease to form spontaneous leptomeningeal collaterals,[28] and are particularly useful in the pediatric population that have increased angioplasticity and vessels too small for an effective direct bypass.

In 1977, Karasawa and colleagues[29] developed EMS for patients in whom an adequate STA was unavailable for bypass, and found favorable results when this indirect measure was performed in 10 patients. Similar to most other techniques, a frontotemporal craniotomy and dural opening is made while preserving the middle meningeal

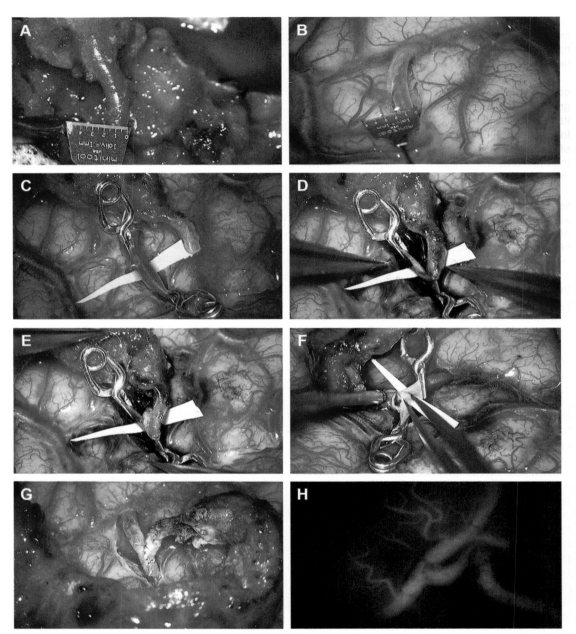

Fig. 3. Intraoperative STA-MCA bypass. (*A*) The STA should be at least 0.8 mm in diameter to achieve an adequate anastomosis. (*B*) After wide opening of the arachnoid, a recipient M4 branch is chosen and used as the recipient vessel. (*C*) Using low profile Lazic (Peter Lazic GmbH, Tuttlingen, Germany) 3-mm temporary clips, the M4 vessel is temporarily occluded. (*D*) An elliptical arteriotomy is made in the recipient vessel. Methylene blue or indigo carmine dye is then applied to the M4 vessel to improve visualization. The toe of the fishmouthed STA is sutured first using 10 to 0 Monosof (Convidien, Mansfield, MA) suture. (*E*) The heel of the STA is then sutured. (*F*) The side walls are sutured using 10 to 0 Monosof sutures, ensuring not to catch the back wall of the recipient vessel. (*G*) Once the anastomosis is completed, the STA and its vascular cuff are placed onto the cortical surface. (*H*) ICG video angiography is used to confirm patency of the anastomosis. (*From* Gooderham P, Steinberg GK. Intracranial-Extracranial Bypass surgery for Moyamoya Disease. In: Spetzler M, Kalani Y, Nakaji P, editors. Neurovascular Surgery 2nd Edition. New York: Thieme; 2015(95). p. 1156–71. with permission.)

artery. Placement of the temporalis muscle directly over the brain surface is performed followed by suturing of the muscle edges to the remaining dural leaflets.[29]

EDAS was first described by Matsushima and colleagues in 1981[30] who noted successful angiographic outcomes with EMS yet wanted to avoid its associated complications (temporary neurologic deterioration and focal seizures). Movement of the temporalis muscle directly in contact with the brain was also seen as a potential adverse effect on the underlying brain.

EDAS as described by Matsushima and colleagues[30] involves isolating a scalp artery of interest followed by creation of a 5-mm to 7-mm strip of galeal cuff attached to the donor artery. Once separated from the underlying periosteum and temporalis fascia, the muscle is opened and a craniotomy is performed. A vertical incision is then made in the dura, with careful attention not to coagulate or cut large middle meningeal vessels that can provide another means of revascularization. The arachnoid was left intact based on the notion that cerebrospinal fluid between the brain and donor vessel would hinder collateral formation. The galeal cuff is then sutured to the dural edges in a watertight fashion.

At our institution, EDAS is the procedure of choice when an indirect graft is chosen. In contrast to Matsushima and colleagues,[30] the senior author opens the arachnoid widely and lays the STA with its vascular cuff directly onto the brain pial surface without suturing to the dura or pia. Although variations of EDAS have evolved over time among different groups, all techniques share the same principle of delayed collateral formation between the STA and its associated vascularized tissue and the underlying brain. A slight modification to the EDAS procedure using pial synangiosis was popularized by Scott and colleagues.[31] When pial synangiosis is performed, the STA is sutured to the underlying pia using 10–0 monofilament after the arachnoid is widely opened.

Another variation to EDAS, split DES, uses the inner layer of the dura to expand the area of revascularization potential. This technique, described by Kashiwagi and colleagues in Japan, uses the standard EDAS followed by an H-shaped incision that splits the outer layer of the dura only and leaves the inner dural leaflet intact.[32] Careful attention is made not to injure the anterior or posterior branches of the middle meningeal artery. The inner dural layer is then similarly cut, folded, and tucked into the subdural space directly onto the cortical surface. Minimal electrocautery of the dura should be used, while using oxycellulose agents to achieve hemostasis. The outer dural layer can then be closed.

By combining EDAS and EMS, Kinugasa created EDAMS for patients lacking appropriate scalp arteries for anastomosis or when more blood flow is desired.[33] This technique takes advantage of the vascularized temporalis muscle along with the meninges and STA to create anastomoses with the cortical surface. Once the arachnoid is widely opened, the STA and folded dural edges are placed in direct contact with the brain surface. The pedicled temporalis muscle can then be positioned over the brain surface and affixed to the surrounding dural edges.

The vast majority of revascularization techniques aim to increase blood flow to the MCA territory. To address the anterior cerebral artery (ACA) territory, which is equally as prone to ischemia,[34] Kinugasa developed ribbon EDAMS to help revascularize the medial frontal lobes.[35] This technique involves tucking a "ribbon" of galea and periosteum cut in a zigzag pattern into the bilateral interhemispheric fissures.

A less technically demanding revascularization strategy is through the use of multiple strategically placed burr holes. This was first recognized when there was evidence of neovascularization at prior ventriculostomy sites.[36] Sainte-Rose and colleagues[37] reviewed their experience using this method in 14 children with moyamoya disease. The surgical technique involved placement of 10 to 24 burr holes over the frontoparietal region followed by both dural and arachnoid opening. This method was found to be both effective and safe and can be considered as the sole treatment in select patients.

INDIRECT TECHNIQUES USING DISTANT TISSUE

Even with the already described indirect and direct techniques, additional revascularization may be necessary in particular circumstances, such as when patients have remote ischemic strokes away from the area of previous revascularization, insufficient collateral formation, or occlusion of a previously used donor vessel. If all donor vessels and adjacent tissue options have been exhausted from prior surgeries, omental transposition can be used as a salvage option (**Fig. 4**). This method of revascularization was first used by Karasawa and colleagues in 1980.[38]

The inherent angiogenic and healing properties of the omentum makes it an excellent source for revascularization when placed over the brain surface. Its ability to stimulate underlying revascularization derives from its high levels of vascular endothelial growth factor protein and other growth/angiogenic factors especially in the presence of hypoxia. The

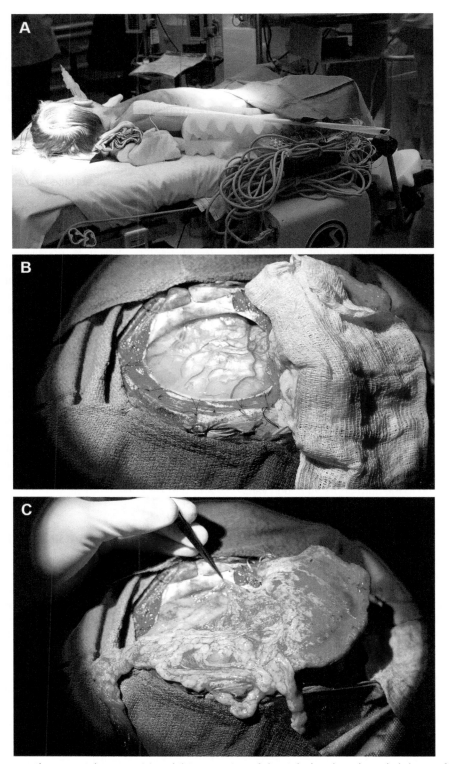

Fig. 4. Intraoperative omental transposition. (*A*) Preparation of the right head, neck, and abdomen for omental bypass (*B*) A large craniotomy and wide dural opening is made to maximize revascularization potential (*C*) The pedicled omentum is tunneled toward the head and placed directly over the brain surface (not shown is drilling of the inner table of the craniotomy flap to accommodate the omental flap). (*From* Navarro R, Chao K, Gooderham PA, et al. Less invasive pedicled omental-cranial transposition in pediatric patients with moyamoya disease and failed prior revascularization. Neurosurgery 2014;10(Suppl 1):1–14; with permission.)

omentum has been widely used by general surgeons for its wound-healing capabilities when treating large open sternotomy wounds, perforated viscus, and obliteration of bronchopleural fistulas.[39]

Historically, omental harvesting has required a large laparotomy with subcutaneous tunneling of the pedicled graft to the craniotomy. When an open laparotomy is performed, complication rates as high as 18.5% have been reported, consisting of fascial dehiscence, wound infection, ventral hernia, and postoperative ileus. Due to the morbidity associated with open abdominal procedures, we have described the same omental harvesting using a laparoscopic approach. Between 2011 and 2016, 15 patients with moyamoya disease (7 children, 8 adults) underwent laparoscopic omental cerebral transposition at our institution with the assistance of general surgery. One patient sustained colonic injury intraoperatively and 1 patient experienced persistent omental hernia at the fascial defect postoperatively. All patients had complete symptomatic resolution or improvement of preoperative transient ischemic attacks at follow-up with adequate angiographic revascularization (**Fig. 5**). It should be noted that in some of the patients, the donor omental gastroepiploic artery was not well visualized on 6-month postoperative angiogram, but by parasitizing chest wall and cervical blood supply, maintained robust revascularization of the brain.[39]

The surgical technique requires the neurosurgeon and general surgeon to work together. Although the temporoparietal craniotomy is being made, the general surgeon insufflates the abdomen followed by insertion of a 10-mm, 30-degree telescope into an umbilical incision. Two 5-mm ports are then inserted in the mid-clavicular lines of the upper quadrants. All omental attachments to the colon and splenic region are released, taking extra care to preserve the gastroepiploic vessels that traverse adjacent the greater curvature of the stomach. Once freed, the omentum can be delivered out of the abdominal cavity through another midline incision approximately 2 cm below the xiphoid process. Another skip incision is made superior to the clavicle on the side of the craniotomy. Then using a combination of Pean clamps and lighted retractors, a presternal subcutaneous tract is created between the epigastric and neck incisions. Using a similar technique, a subcutaneous conduit is also made between the craniotomy and supraclavicular incision. By creating a passageway of at least 1 inch in width, the omentum can be passed cephalad largely unobstructed. A silk suture is then tied to the end of the omental flap and tunneled through the subcutaneous space ensuring torsion of the flap does not occur. Once the omentum is at the craniotomy site, the dura and arachnoid are opened widely, allowing for direct contact of the omentum with the underlying pia.

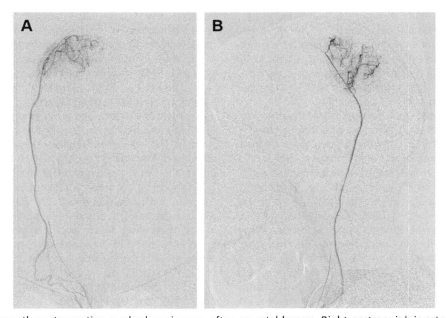

Fig. 5. Six-month postoperative cerebral angiogram after omental bypass. Right gastroepiploic artery injection with anteroposterior (AP) (*A*) and lateral (*B*) projections. Hypertrophy and patency of the gastroepiploic artery with indirect collateral formation to the brain is shown in the parietal area. (*From* Navarro R, Chao K, Gooderham PA, et al. Less invasive pedicled omental-cranial transposition in pediatric patients with moyamoya disease and failed prior revascularization. Neurosurgery 2014;10(Suppl 1):1–14; with permission.)

The omentum is further secured by suturing it to the dural edges.

Although we demonstrated the feasibility of this procedure laparoscopically, the inherent risks of the graft, mass effect from the overlying omentum, risk of torsion, and necrosis, are not negated by this minimally invasive modification.[40] Even though the morbidity involved in open laparotomies can be avoided, this technique is reserved for patients with moyamoya disease who have exhausted all other revascularization possibilities.

Touho and colleagues[41] described gracilis muscle transplantation to the ACA and posterior cerebral artery (PCA) territories in patients who demonstrated decreased blood flow over the frontal or occipital lobes. Although this technique may be successful in a subgroup of patients, we do not routinely perform it at our institution.

DISCUSSION
Benefits of Revascularization

Although there is no randomized controlled trial that confirms the benefit of surgical revascularization in patients presenting with cerebral ischemia, there is compelling evidence among many large case series that surgical revascularization using direct or indirect methods benefit patients with moyamoya disease and helps prevent future risk of ischemic strokes.[16,18,31,42] The high risk of recurrent strokes in patients who are medically treated suggests that surgery is beneficial to patients with moyamoya disease. A 5-year 65% risk of recurrent stroke in patients treated without surgery and an even more compelling 5-year 82% risk of stroke in patients with bilateral disease substantiates the dismal prognosis without cerebral revascularization.[14]

The evidence supporting the benefits of bypass surgery in reducing the risk of recurrent hemorrhage in patients with moyamoya disease has been less compelling until recently. Similar to ischemic strokes, a poor prognosis is also seen in patients with moyamoya disease presenting with hemorrhage, with re-hemorrhage rates as high as 27.8% with a 5.6% mortality after the first bleed.[43] A long-awaited prospective, randomized, controlled trial was conducted in Japan to help elucidate the appropriate management of patients presenting with hemorrhage. Miyamoto and colleagues[12] demonstrated significantly lower rates of recurrent hemorrhage, as well as decreased risk of combined primary endpoint including recurrent hemorrhage, ischemic stroke and crescendo transient ischemic attack (TIA) requiring bypass, and reduced risk of secondary endpoint (reduced recurrent hemorrhage and death/severe disability) in patients undergoing *direct* bypass when compared with conservative management. Chronic hemodynamic stress on moyamoya collateral vessels has been implicated as the cause of hemorrhage in these patients. Moyamoya vessels have been shown to angiographically disappear after bypass surgery, presumably due to the offloaded hemodynamic stress.[44] This phenomenon was reported at our institution in a 5-year-old boy who demonstrated rapid near complete resolution of angiographic moyamoya vessels after bilateral STA/MCA bypasses with concurrent unilateral EDAS.[45]

Direct Versus Indirect Bypass and Outcomes

There is currently no randomized controlled trial that clearly demonstrates one technique (indirect, direct, combined) is more efficacious than another in the treatment of moyamoya disease. Direct comparison between the 2 techniques is difficult and unreliable, as many direct anastomoses reported in the literature inevitably integrate an indirect method of revascularization, and hence a combined technique. Although more technically demanding and time-consuming, many investigators have suggested that direct bypass is superior to indirect techniques due to the immediate increase in blood flow to the brain, more consistent angiographic neovascularization over time, and ability to restore normal hemodynamic reserve on cerebral blood flow (CBF) studies, as well as reduced risk of recurrent TIAs and recurrent stroke, particularly in adult moyamoya patients.[44,46-53]

Miyamoto and colleagues[54] analyzed the clinical course of 113 patients with moyamoya disease who underwent direct STA-MCA anastomosis with or without EDAMS for up to 24 years. Of the 113 patients, 110 stopped experiencing ischemic episodes and 100 patients eventually returned to normal daily living. Ishikawa and colleagues[48] similarly demonstrated the efficacy of direct revascularization in the prevention of ischemic events by comparing a combined (direct/indirect) STA-MCA bypass and EDAMS with EDAMS alone. The incidence of postoperative ischemic attacks in the combined group and the indirect group were 10% and 56%, respectively. Thus, ischemic attacks were significantly less in the combined group ($P<.01$).[48]

At our institution, the senior author performs combined (direct/indirect) bypasses for symptomatic patients with occlusion of the ICA or MCA with poor cerebrovascular reserve. Special consideration is given to patients with occlusive disease who have robust collateral formation on preoperative angiography with rapid retrograde filling of the

ICA or MCA territory in conjunction with normal intraoperative blood flow measurements of the recipient artery. In these instances, an indirect bypass may be chosen because additional immediate blood flow is not required.

At Stanford, we have performed more than 1446 bypasses in more than 905 patients for moyamoya disease. Traditionally, our practice has been to perform a direct bypass when technically feasible. Over time, the STA can hypertrophy to meet the oxygen demands of the brain and provide more consistent collateral formation on follow-up angiography, with the added benefit of providing immediate augmented blood flow (**Fig. 6**). The invested vascularized galeal cuff on the donor artery also provides additional indirect collaterals that form

over time. In our published series of 557 surgeries (389 adults and 168 pediatric), a direct bypass was used in 95.1% of adult and 76.2% of pediatric patients. At a mean follow-up of 1.5 years, 99% of the bypasses were angiographically patent. The rare cases with occluded bypasses were still able to develop indirect collaterals with the underlying brain. Outcome analysis was performed on 264 patients (450 surgeries) based on a minimum of 6 months of follow-up. Within this cohort, a significant neurologic deficit occurred in 3.5% of procedures or 5.6% of patients. Of 264 patients, 3.0% (8 patients) sustained ischemic strokes in either the ipsilateral (4 patients) or contralateral (4 patients) hemisphere and 2.6% (7 patients) suffered a new postoperative hemorrhage. The cumulative

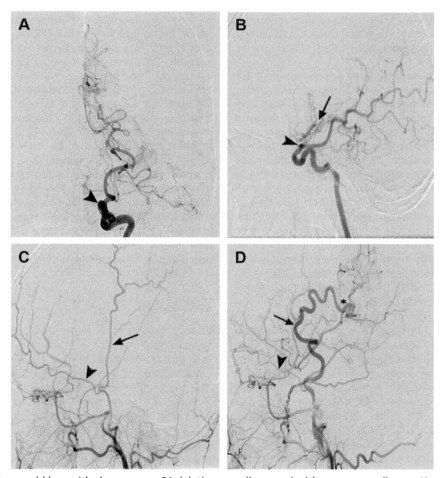

Fig. 6. A 13-year-old boy with chromosome 21 deletion was diagnosed with moyamoya disease. He underwent a left direct STA-MCA bypass. Preoperative cerebral angiogram, ICA injection, and AP and lateral views (*A* and *B*, respectively) showing ICA occlusion (*arrowhead*) just distal to the posterior communicating artery and moyamoya vessels formation (*arrow*). (*C*) Lateral projection of the preoperative STA showing both parietal (*arrow*) and frontal (*arrowhead*) branches. (*D*) Three-year postoperative angiogram showing a widely patent anastomosis (*asterisk*) with hypertrophy of the parietal STA donor vessel (*arrow*). Frontal STA branch shown for size comparison (*arrowhead*).

5-year risk of stroke or death was 5.5%, which compares favorably to the natural history of moyamoya disease if left untreated. Long-term outcomes also portended a favorable course with improvements in the frequency of TIAs, headaches, and in Modified Rankin Scale (mRS) from 1.62 preoperatively to 0.83 (P<.0001) at a mean follow-up of 4.9 years. At Stanford, from 1991 to 2014, for 1244 bypass procedures in 765 patients with moyamoya disease, the rate of repeat revascularization for recurrent symptoms after previous direct bypass was 1% versus 4% if a prior indirect procedure was performed initially (P = .03), An indirect bypass is reserved for children younger than 4 years old; patients with severe stenosis of ICA or MCA with preserved orthograde blood flow, but not complete occlusion; or when the donor or recipient vessels are too small to perform an anastomosis (<0.8 mm).[16] Repeat revascularization in a different vascular territory not adequately addressed by the prior procedure may also require an indirect graft.

Indirect bypasses have the added benefit of not requiring temporary occlusion of an M4 branch, which is necessary in direct bypasses. Scott and colleagues[31] showed the success of indirect bypass in pediatric patients using pial synangiosis in a large, single-institution experience. In 143 pediatric patients undergoing pial synangiosis, most of these treated children stopped experiencing strokes and TIAs, with 75% of children leading independent lives at 1 year follow-up.[31] Starke and colleagues[51] performed EDAS in 43 adult patients with moyamoya disease (67 hemispheres) and demonstrated a 5-year ipsilateral stroke rate of 6% versus 64% in the contralateral, nonoperated side. Dusick and colleagues[50] showed that indirect bypass using EDAS and multiple burr holes effectively provided 95% prevention of recurrent ischemia or hemorrhage in adults and children, although median follow-up was only 14 months.

Recently, Kazumata and colleagues[46] performed a systematic review of 35 studies including 2032 direct bypasses and 4171 indirect revascularization procedures. Postoperative stroke rates were found to be 5.4% (95% confidence interval [CI] 3.4%–7.5%) in the direct/combined group and 5.5% (95% CI 3.7%–7.3%) in the indirect group per surgery. Recurrent stroke rates were found to be 3.5% for in the direct/combined bypass group compared with 11.2% for patients undergoing indirect procedures (P<.05) with mean follow-up of 4 years, suggesting direct bypass was superior to indirect in preventing future recurrent strokes.

Alternatively, a recent retrospective comparative effectiveness analysis of 33 studies consisting of 4197 moyamoya cases demonstrated that indirect procedures were superior to direct in terms of quality-adjusted life years; however, it is not clear how clinically meaningful this would be for patients[53]

We believe performing direct bypasses in noncompletely occluded ICA or MCA moyamoya disease may compete with the native flow or accelerate secondary occlusion of an already stenotic ICA or MCA. Indirect grafts are chosen in these circumstances especially if immediate increased blood flow is not needed. Final decisions to proceed with an entirely indirect revascularization are based on preoperative angiography, cerebrovascular reserve, and intraoperative blood flow measurements of the recipient M4 branch.

As mean flow across a microanastomosis site in the M4 recipient can increase as much as fivefold after direct bypass,[55] a paradoxic competition in blood flow may occur between the site of anastomosis and the abnormal native vascular network. This phenomenon may promote stasis with local increased ischemia or subsequent occlusion of an already stenosed ICA or MCA. Although not in patients with moyamoya disease, this potential complication has been observed in patients undergoing STA-MCA bypass for atherosclerotic intracranial stenosis in which the native circulation thrombosed and occluded a few days after bypass with subsequent ischemic strokes.[56] The method of revascularization (direct/indirect) in patients with arterial stenosis without occlusion, therefore, require special attention, as immediately augmenting flow may adversely alter underlying hemodynamic parameters and lead to preventable perioperative strokes and morbidity.

SUMMARY

The management of moyamoya disease is not only unique, but also a practice that continues to evolve. At our institution, we have used a combined approach with excellent clinical success. This approach provides a direct anastomosis that supplies immediate augmented blood flow, while also taking advantage of indirect collaterals that form over time. However, we believe a subgroup of patients with ICA or MCA stenosis but not complete occlusion deserves special consideration for an entirely indirect bypass when immediate augmented blood flow is not needed. The surgical management of patients with moyamoya disease has proven to be complex and should remain individually tailored to address the patient's symptoms, risk of future stroke, and blood flow requirements of the patient.

REFERENCES

1. Takeuchi K, Shimizu K. Hypoplasia of the bilateral internal carotid arteries. Brain Nerve 1957;9:37–43.
2. Suzuki J, Takaku A. Cerebrovascular "moyamoya" disease. Disease showing abnormal net-like vessels in base of brain. Arch Neurol 1969;20(3):288–99.
3. Yamauchi T, Houkin K, Tada M, et al. Familial occurrence of moyamoya disease. Clin Neurol Neurosurg 1997;99(Suppl 2):S162–7.
4. Starke RM, Crowley RW, Maltenfort M, et al. Moyamoya disorder in the United States. Neurosurgery 2012;71(1):93–9.
5. Uchino K, Johnston SC, Becker KJ, et al. Moyamoya disease in Washington State and California. Neurology 2005;65(6):956–8.
6. Kuriyama S, Kusaka Y, Fujimura M, et al. Prevalence and clinicoepidemiological features of moyamoya disease in Japan: findings from a nationwide epidemiological survey. Stroke 2008;39(1):42–7.
7. Fukui M, Kono S, Sueishi K, et al. Moyamoya disease. Neuropathology 2000;20(Suppl):S61–4.
8. Houkin K, Yoshimoto T, Abe H, et al. Role of basic fibroblast growth factor in the pathogenesis of moyamoya disease. Neurosurg Focus 1998;5(5):e2.
9. Oka K, Yamashita M, Sadoshima S, et al. Cerebral haemorrhage in Moyamoya disease at autopsy. Virchows Arch A Pathol Anat Histol 1981;392(3):247–61.
10. Yamashita M, Oka K, Tanaka K. Histopathology of the brain vascular network in moyamoya disease. Stroke 1983;14(1):50–8.
11. Nishimoto A. Moyamoya disease (author's transl). Neurol Med Chir (Tokyo) 1979;19(3):221–8 [in Japanese].
12. Miyamoto S, Yoshimoto T, Hashimoto N, et al. Effects of extracranial-intracranial bypass for patients with hemorrhagic moyamoya disease: results of the Japan Adult Moyamoya Trial. Stroke 2014;45(5):1415–21.
13. Kraemer M, Heienbrok W, Berlit P. Moyamoya disease in Europeans. Stroke 2008;39(12):3193–200.
14. Hallemeier CL, Rich KM, Grubb RL Jr, et al. Clinical features and outcome in North American adults with moyamoya phenomenon. Stroke 2006;37(6):1490–6.
15. Numaguchi Y, Gonzalez CF, Davis PC, et al. Moyamoya disease in the United States. Clin Neurol Neurosurg 1997;99(Suppl 2):S26–30.
16. Guzman R, Lee M, Achrol A, et al. Clinical outcome after 450 revascularization procedures for moyamoya disease. Clinical article. J Neurosurg 2009;111(5):927–35.
17. Antonucci MU, Burns TC, Pulling TM, et al. Acute preoperative infarcts and poor cerebrovascular reserve are independent risk factors for severe ischemic complications following direct extracranial-intracranial bypass for moyamoya disease. AJNR Am J Neuroradiol 2016;37(2):228–35.
18. Fung LW, Thompson D, Ganesan V. Revascularisation surgery for paediatric moyamoya: a review of the literature. Childs Nerv Syst 2005;21(5):358–64.
19. Choi JU, Kim DS, Kim EY, et al. Natural history of moyamoya disease: comparison of activity of daily living in surgery and non surgery groups. Clin Neurol Neurosurg 1997;99(Suppl 2):S11–8.
20. Kuroda S, Ishikawa T, Houkin K, et al. Incidence and clinical features of disease progression in adult moyamoya disease. Stroke 2005;36(10):2148–53.
21. Kurokawa T, Tomita S, Ueda K, et al. Prognosis of occlusive disease of the circle of Willis (moyamoya disease) in children. Pediatr Neurol 1985;1(5):274–7.
22. Kuroda S, Hashimoto N, Yoshimoto T, et al. Research Committee on Moyamoya Disease in Japan. Radiological findings, clinical course, and outcome in asymptomatic moyamoya disease: results of multicenter survey in Japan. Stroke 2007;38(5):1430–5.
23. Gross BA, Du R. The natural history of moyamoya in a North American adult cohort. J Clin Neurosci 2013;20(1):44–8.
24. McLean MJ, Gebarski SS, van der Spek AF, et al. Response of moyamoya disease to verapamil. Lancet 1985;1(8421):163–4.
25. Khan N, Dodd R, Marks MP, et al. Failure of primary percutaneous angioplasty and stenting in the prevention of ischemia in Moyamoya angiopathy. Cerebrovasc Dis 2011;31(2):147–53.
26. Kikuchi H, Karasawa J. [STA-cortical MCA anastomosis for cerebrovascular occlusive disease.] No Shinkei Geka 1:15-19, 1973 (Jpn)
27. Pandey P, Steinberg GK. Neurosurgical advances in the treatment of moyamoya disease. Stroke 2011;42(11):3304–10.
28. Matsushima T, Fukui M, Kitamura K, et al. Encephalo-duro-arterio-synangiosis in children with moyamoya disease. Acta Neurochir (Wien) 1990;104(3–4):96–102.
29. Karasawa J, Kikuchi H, Furuse S, et al. A surgical treatment of "moyamoya" disease "encephalo-myo synangiosis". Neurol Med Chir (Tokyo) 1977;17(1 Pt 1):29–37.
30. Matsushima Y, Fukai N, Tanaka K, et al. A new surgical treatment of moyamoya disease in children: a preliminary report. Surg Neurol 1981;15(4):313–20.
31. Scott RM, Smith JL, Robertson RL, et al. Long-term outcome in children with moyamoya syndrome after cranial revascularization by pial synangiosis. J Neurosurg 2004;100(2 Suppl Pediatrics):142–9.
32. Kashiwagi S, Kato S, Yamashita K, et al. Revascularization with split duro-encephalo-synangiosis in the pediatric moyamoya disease–surgical result and clinical outcome. Clin Neurol Neurosurg 1997;99(Suppl 2):S115–7.
33. Kinugasa K, Mandai S, Kamata I, et al. Surgical treatment of moyamoya disease: operative technique for encephalo-duro-arterio-myo-synangiosis,

its follow-up, clinical results, and angiograms. Neurosurgery 1993;32(4):527–31.

34. Suzuki R, Matsushima Y, Takada Y, et al. Changes in cerebral hemodynamics following encephalo-duro-arterio-synangiosis (EDAS) in young patients with moyamoya disease. Surg Neurol 1989;31(5): 343–9.

35. Kinugasa K, Mandai S, Tokunaga K, et al. Ribbon enchephalo-duro-arterio-myo-synangiosis for moyamoya disease. Surg Neurol 1994;41(6):455–61.

36. Endo M, Kawano N, Miyaska Y, et al. Cranial burr hole for revascularization in moyamoya disease. J Neurosurg 1989;71(2):180–5.

37. Sainte-Rose C, Oliveira R, Puget S, et al. Multiple bur hole surgery for the treatment of moyamoya disease in children. J Neurosurg 2006;105(6 Suppl): 437–43.

38. Karasawa J, Kikuchi H, Kawamura J, et al. Intracranial transplantation of the omentum for cerebrovascular moyamoya disease: a two-year follow-up study. Surg Neurol 1980;14(6):444–9.

39. Bruzoni M, Steinberg GK, Dutta S. Laparoscopic harvesting of omental pedicle flap for cerebral revascularization in children with moyamoya disease. J Pediatr Surg 2016;51(4):592–7.

40. Navarro R, Chao K, Gooderham PA, et al. Less invasive pedicled omental-cranial transposition in pediatric patients with moyamoya disease and failed prior revascularization. Neurosurgery 2014;10(Suppl 1): 1–14.

41. Touho H, Karasawa J, Ohnishi H. Cerebral revascularization using gracilis muscle transplantation for childhood moyamoya disease. Surg Neurol 1995; 43(2):191–7 [discussion: 197–8].

42. Nakashima H, Meguro T, Kawada S, et al. Long-term results of surgically treated moyamoya disease. Clin Neurol Neurosurg 1997;99(Suppl 2):S156–61.

43. Saeki N, Yamaura A, Hoshi S, et al. Hemorrhagic type of moyamoya disease. No Shinkei Geka 1991; 19(8):705–12 [in Japanese].

44. Houkin K, Kamiyama H, Abe H, et al. Surgical therapy for adult moyamoya disease. Can surgical revascularization prevent the recurrence of intracerebral hemorrhage? Stroke 1996;27(8):1342–6.

45. Wang MY, Steinberg GK. Rapid and near-complete resolution of moyamoya vessels in a patient with moyamoya disease treated with superficial temporal artery-middle cerebral artery bypass. Pediatr Neurosurg 1996;24(3):145–50.

46. Kazumata K, Ito M, Tokairin K, et al. The frequency of postoperative stroke in moyamoya disease following combined revascularization: a single-university series and systematic review. J Neurosurg 2014; 121(2):432–40.

47. Mizoi K, Kayama T, Yoshimoto T, et al. Indirect revascularization for moyamoya disease: is there a beneficial effect for adult patients? Surg Neurol 1996; 45(6):541–8 [discussion: 548–9].

48. Ishikawa T, Houkin K, Kamiyama H, et al. Effects of surgical revascularization on outcome of patients with pediatric moyamoya disease. Stroke 1997;28(6): 1170–3.

49. Agarwalla PK, Stapleton CJ, Phillips MT, et al. Surgical outcomes following encephaloduroarteriosynangiosis in North American adults with moyamoya. J Neurosurg 2014;121(6):1394–400.

50. Dusick JR, Gonzalez NR, Martin NA. Clinical and angiographic outcomes from indirect revascularization surgery for Moyamoya disease in adults and children: a review of 63 procedures. Neurosurgery 2011;68(1):34–43 [discussion: 43].

51. Starke RM, Komotar RJ, Hickman ZL, et al. Clinical features, surgical treatment, and long-term outcome in adult patients with moyamoya disease. Clinical article. J Neurosurg 2009;111(5):936–42.

52. Veeravagu A, Guzman R, Patil CG, et al. Moyamoya disease in pediatric patients: outcomes of neurosurgical interventions. Neurosurg Focus 2008; 24(2):E16.

53. Macyszyn L, Attiah M, Ma TS, et al. Direct versus indirect revascularization procedures for moyamoya disease: a comparative effectiveness study. J Neurosurg 2016;1–7.

54. Miyamoto S, Akiyama Y, Nagata I, et al. Long-term outcome after STA-MCA anastomosis for moyamoya disease. Neurosurg Focus 1998;5(5):e5.

55. Lee M, Guzman R, Bell-Stephens T, et al. Intraoperative blood flow analysis of direct revascularization procedures in patients with moyamoya disease. J Cereb Blood Flow Metab 2011;31(1):262–74.

56. Awad I, Furlan AJ, Little JR. Changes in intracranial stenotic lesions after extracranial-intracranial bypass surgery. J Neurosurg 1984;60(4):771–6.

Flow Diversion after Aneurysmal Subarachnoid Hemorrhage

Sabareesh K. Natarajan, MD, MS[a,b,c,d,g,h], Hussain Shallwani, MD[a,b,c,d,g,h],
Vernard S. Fennell, MD, MSc[a,b,c,d,g,h], Jeffrey S. Beecher, DO[a,b,c,d,g,h],
Hakeem J. Shakir, MD[a,b,c,d,e,f,g,h], Jason M. Davies, MD, PhD[a,b,c,d,e,f,g,h],
Kenneth V. Snyder, MD, PhD[a,b,c,d,f,g,h], Adnan H. Siddiqui, MD, PhD[a,b,c,d,e,f],
Elad I. Levy, MD, MBA[f,g,h],*

KEYWORDS

- Cerebral aneurysm • Flow diversion • Pipeline Embolization Device • Subarachnoid hemorrhage

KEY POINTS

- Flow diversion is not the primary treatment of choice after aneurysmal subarachnoid hemorrhage (SAH) but is a reasonable final option if other, safer options are not available to treat the aneurysm.
- In the setting of acute aneurysm rupture, protection of the aneurysm dome by traditional endovascular or microsurgical means followed by delayed flow diversion is a safer choice than primary flow diversion.
- Our experience and review of the literature show the feasibility of flow diversion in the setting of acute rupture either as primary treatment or in a subacute fashion after dome protection.
- Careful patient selection, selective use of coiling, timing of flow diversion after dome protection, and the timing of heparin and antiplatelet therapy in the periprocedural period improve the safety of flow diversion as a strategy in aneurysmal SAH.
- Shield technology may decrease the duration and/or the need for dual antiplatelet therapy, thereby making flow diversion safer in the setting of aneurysm rupture.

INTERNATIONAL SUBARACHNOID ANEURYSM TRIAL ESTABLISHED ENDOVASCULAR TREATMENT AS THE PRIMARY TREATMENT OF RUPTURED ANEURYSMS

The International Subarachnoid Aneurysm Trial (ISAT) established endovascular treatment as the primary modality of treatment in patients with aneurysmal subarachnoid hemorrhage (SAH) if there was clear equipoise between both surgical clipping and endovascular coiling.[1] The ISAT investigators randomized 2143 patients to clipping versus coiling and found an absolute risk reduction of approximately 7% in death or dependency at 1 year with coiling. Patients in the endovascular

Disclosure: See last page of article.
[a] Department of Neurosurgery, Jacobs School of Medicine and Biomedical Sciences, University at Buffalo, State University of New York, 100 High Street, Buffalo, NY 14203, USA; [b] Gates Vascular Institute, Kaleida Health, 100 High Street, Buffalo, NY 14203, USA; [c] University at Buffalo, State University of New York, 875 Ellicott Street, 5th Floor, Buffalo, NY 14203, USA; [d] Neurosurgical Stroke Service, Kaleida Health, 100 High Street, Buffalo, NY 14203, USA; [e] The Jacobs Institute, 875 Ellicott Street, 5th Floor, Buffalo, NY 14203, USA; [f] Toshiba Stroke & Vascular Research Center, University at Buffalo, State University of New York, 875 Ellicott Street, Buffalo, NY 14214, USA; [g] Jacobs School of Medicine and Biomedical Sciences, University at Buffalo, State University of New York, 3435 Main Street, Buffalo, NY 14214, USA; [h] Neuroendovascular Services, Gates Vascular Institute, Kaleida Health, Buffalo, 100 High Street, Buffalo, NY, USA
* Corresponding author. Attention: Editorial Office, University at Buffalo Neurosurgery, 100 High Street, Suite B4, Buffalo, NY 14203.
E-mail address: elevy@ubns.com

neurosurgery.theclinics.com

treatment group were more likely to be alive and independent at 10 years than were patients in the neurosurgery group (odds ratio [OR], 1·34; 95% confidence interval [CI], 1·07–1·67). Thirty-three patients had a recurrent SAH more than 1 year after their initial hemorrhage (in 17, the SAH was from rupture of the target aneurysm).[2,3] Rebleeding was more likely after endovascular coiling (1 in 641 patient years; 0.15%) than after neurosurgical clipping (1 in 2041 patient years; 0.05%), but the risk was small in both groups.

WHO GETS CLIPPED AFTER THE INTERNATIONAL SUBARACHNOID ANEURYSM TRIAL?

The presence of subarachnoid blood and brain edema in the acute phase of SAH makes surgical dissection difficult but does not affect the technique of endovascular (endosaccular) coiling. Patients who have been treated preferentially by clipping after the ISAT are those who could not safely undergo endovascular therapies, such as patients with wide-necked or fusiform aneurysms with branch incorporation at the neck or middle cerebral artery (MCA) bifurcation aneurysms, or younger patients with good Hunt and Hess grades (1–3) who would benefit from a theoretically more durable treatment in the long run.

ENDOVASCULAR DEVICES ARE DEVELOPING AT A RAPID PACE TO ENABLE TREATMENT OF MORE COMPLEX ANEURYSM MORPHOLOGIES AND TO DECREASE RECURRENCE RATES

Nevertheless, the permanent aneurysm occlusion rate after simple primary coiling is only 40% to 45%.[4] Endovascular devices are rapidly being developed and enabling the treatment of wide-necked and complex aneurysms with stent assistance, bifurcation devices, and flow diverters. Stent assistance and the use of flow diverters have increased the durability of endovascular treatments. These developments in endovascular devices and techniques are diminishing the argument that younger patients need to be treated by microsurgical means to achieve long-lasting aneurysm occlusion.

OUR PROTOCOL FOR ANEURYSMAL SUBARACHNOID HEMORRHAGE

At our center, an external ventricular drain (EVD) is placed in patients with aneurysmal SAH who present with Hunt and Hess grades 3 or higher in the emergency room (open to drain at 20 cm above the tragus) after undergoing a non–contrast-enhanced computed tomography (CT) scan of the head. A CT angiogram of the head and neck is obtained after EVD placement. If the CT angiogram shows an aneurysm, a diagnostic cerebral digital subtraction angiogram is performed and plans are made for possible treatment within 24 hours. Until the aneurysm is treated, the patient is monitored in the neurointensive care unit with strict systolic blood pressure control, maintained under 130 mm Hg. The diagnostic angiogram is performed under conscious sedation if the patient is awake unless the patient is uncooperative.

The right femoral artery is accessed with a micropuncture needle. Using a modified Seldinger technique, a 6-French (F) sheath is placed. After performing an angiographic run of the right femoral artery, a 0.89-mm (0.035-inch) Glidewire (Terumo, Somerset, NJ) and a 5-F angled or Simmons II catheter (Terumo) are advanced as a unit to the aortic arch, and the supra-aortic vessels are engaged. Selective catheterization of both internal carotid arteries (ICAs) and the dominant vertebral artery (VA) is performed to obtain optimal images of the entire cerebral circulation. A three-dimensional (3D) rotational angiogram is obtained, and the images are transferred to an external workstation to better appreciate the morphology of the aneurysm, especially the size of the neck and the involvement of branch vessels in the aneurysm neck. Then, we select orthogonal views for microcatheterization of the aneurysm and attempt primary coiling of the aneurysm with or without balloon assistance. The goal of this treatment is primarily dome protection and obliteration of daughter sacs or focal outpouchings (so-called Murphy's tits), which are common rupture points in aneurysms. Patients in whom primary dome protection is not feasible (blister, fusiform, dissecting, or very wide-necked aneurysms) are assessed for their candidacy for microsurgical obliteration of the aneurysm. If the aneurysm morphology is complex (eg, blister or fusiform aneurysms) and/or if the patient is not a good candidate for surgical clipping (eg, elderly patients and/or those with poor Hunt and Hess grades), flow diversion or stent assistance is attempted to achieve aneurysm occlusion.

Patients are observed in the neurointensive care unit for 14 days after securing the aneurysm (by open or endovascular means), focusing on vasospasm management, gradual weaning from the EVD, and rehabilitation. If the patient was treated by endovascular methods, we perform a repeat diagnostic angiogram to assess aneurysm occlusion before discharge. If the aneurysm is not completely occluded at this point, we perform definitive therapy, which could include either further primary coiling with or without balloon assistance, stent-assisted/device-assisted coiling, or flow diversion before the patient is discharged.

WHAT IS FLOW DIVERSION?

Flow diversion is the placement of a low-porosity, high-mesh-density device in the parent vessel at the aneurysm neck to decrease flow into the aneurysm and redirect the flow to the distal part of the parent vessel. This method facilitates endothelialization of the flow-diverting device and subsequently excludes the aneurysm from the circulation over time. The Pipeline Embolization Device (PED; Medtronic, Minneapolis, MN) has been used for flow diversion in most of our patients because it is the only flow diverter approved by the Food and Drug Administration in the United States. The PED is a 48-wire, mesh-braided stent made of a radiolucent cobalt-chromium alloy, with every fourth strand made of radiopaque platinum-tungsten. Current flow diverters necessitate 3 months of dual antiplatelet therapy and lifelong aspirin to avoid in-stent thrombosis.

FLOW DIVERSION IS NOT THE PREFERRED TREATMENT AFTER ANEURYSMAL SUBARACHNOID HEMORRHAGE

Flow diversion after aneurysmal SAH is not preferred as the primary modality of treatment because of the risk associated with dual antiplatelet regimens in the setting of acute rupture. Moreover, the performance of invasive procedures in the preprocedural or periprocedural period, which may include the placement of an EVD, central line, shunt, tracheostomy, and/or percutaneous endoscopic gastrostomy tube, as well as a craniotomy for evacuation of hematoma and decompression, carries additional risk for patients who are receiving dual antiplatelet therapy. In addition, flow diversion does not achieve immediate aneurysm occlusion and does not decrease the chances of immediate rerupture compared with primary coiling or clipping.

PATIENT SELECTION FOR FLOW DIVERSION AFTER ANEURYSMAL SUBARACHNOID HEMORRHAGE

Patients are considered candidates for flow diversion after aneurysmal SAH at our center in the following circumstances: (1) the acute setting, when we cannot achieve dome protection by any other means given the morphology of the aneurysm (ie, dissecting, giant, blister, or fusiform) and if the patient is not a candidate for microsurgical clipping of the aneurysm as determined by

a multidisciplinary team; and (2) for definitive therapy before discharge if aneurysm occlusion is not observed on the follow-up angiogram at discharge (in patients treated with primary or balloon-assisted coiling). Most aneurysms that require flow diversion are in the paraclinoid and communicating segments of the ICA or intracranial VA with or without involvement of the vertebrobasilar junction.

ANTIPLATELET THERAPY

When flow diversion is chosen as the therapy, any required invasive procedures, including the placement of a central line and an EVD, are performed first. The patient then receives a loading dose of 650 mg of aspirin and 600 mg of clopidogrel and the antiplatelet response is checked with Verify-Now assays (Accriva Diagnostics, San Diego, CA). If the patient is not therapeutic (ie, a nonresponder) on aspirin (reaction units value >550), another loading dose of 650 mg of aspirin is administered. If the patient is not therapeutic on clopidogrel (reaction units value ≥200), a loading dose of 180 mg of Brilinta (AstraZeneca, London, United Kingdom) is administered. We check the reaction units' value after administering the Brilinta loading dose to make sure the value is less than 200 before proceeding with flow diversion (we previously used prasugrel, but Brilinta is our current drug of choice for clopidogrel nonresponders). After the procedure, the patient is maintained on aspirin (325 mg daily) for life and clopidogrel (75 mg daily) or Brilinta (90 mg daily) for approximately 3 months.

FLOW-DIVERSION TECHNIQUE

The procedure is performed under conscious sedation if the patient is cooperative. Either a 6-F Envoy DA XB guiding catheter (Codman Neuro, Raynham, MA) or a biaxial system consisting of a 2.24-mm (088-inch) Neuron Max guide (Penumbra Inc, Alameda, CA) and 115-cm Navien 058 intermediate catheter (Medtronic) used for access. The patient is given heparin to maintain an activated coagulation time of greater than 250 seconds after dome protection (if adjunctive coils are used) or after placement of the first PED (if no coils were used; the use of coils and indications for coiling are discussed later). A 150-cm 0.69-mm (0.027-inch) catheter (eg, Marksman [Medtronic], XT-27 [Stryker Neurovascular, Kalamazoo, MI], or Phenom 27 [Medtronic]) is used for microcatheter access distal to the aneurysm with a Synchro 2 wire (Stryker Neurovascular). After distal microcatheter access has been established, the guide system is advanced coaxially as distal as possible to the petrocavernous region or the V4 segment of the VA to provide excellent support for tracking the PED. At that point, the Synchro 2 wire is removed, and a Pipeline Flex device (Medtronic) is loaded in the microcatheter and advanced until the coil tip of the device is just outside the guiding catheter. The redundancy in the microcatheter is reduced by decreasing the slack in the catheter until the catheter tip can be seen moving and the device is then advanced forward. Once the device is distal to the aneurysm, the Envoy DA XB or Navien catheter is coaxially advanced into the posterior genu/horizontal portion of the cavernous sinus or V4 segment of the VA to assist in delivery of the PED from the microcatheter. The coil tip is unsheathed in a straight segment of the cerebral vasculature (commonly in the M1 segment of the MCA). The entire system is retracted with the coil tip unsheathed so that the Pipeline device is just distal to the distal landing zone. The device is then pushed out from the microcatheter. When a sufficient length of the device is exposed, we wait for 1 or 2 minutes to allow the release and expansion of the distal portion of the device to the size of the vessel lumen. The microcatheter is carefully moved from side to side to assist in the release and opening of the distal end of the device. The device is then carefully delivered from the microcatheter using a push-pull technique, while maintaining wall apposition through the entire length of the device and avoiding kinks around turns in the parent vessel. The last part of the device is typically unsheathed and not pushed out so that the resheathing pad is released from the microcatheter and the device comes free. At this point, the microcatheter is brought back over the deployment mechanism to catch the distal end of the Pipeline device and compact the device. The Envoy DA XB or Navien can also brought up to catch the proximal portion of the device and assist in compacting the device. The entire delivery system with the microcatheter is withdrawn, and final runs are obtained.

OUR EXPERIENCE WITH FLOW DIVERSION AFTER SUBARACHNOID HEMORRHAGE

Eleven patients with 14 aneurysms underwent flow diversion in the acute setting after presenting with SAH at our center between July 2011 and June 2016 (University at Buffalo Institutional Review Board Project MOD00001046). Some of these patients were included in the series reported by Lin and colleagues[5] and/or Linfante and colleagues.[6] There were 8 women and 3 men, with a mean age of 52 ± 13.7 years. The median time from

presentation to treatment was 1 day (range, 0–13 days). Eleven aneurysms were located in the anterior circulation (ICA), whereas 3 were located in the posterior circulation (2 in the VA and 1 in the basilar artery [BA]). The mean greatest dimension of the aneurysm was 5 ± 5.3 mm. The shapes of these aneurysms were saccular in 5, blister in 6, fusiform in 1, and dissecting in 2. Two aneurysms had been coiled previously for dome protection. Flow diversion alone was performed for treatment in all cases, except case 11, for which coils were used to support the PED spanning the patient's fusiform aneurysm. Only 1 PED was deployed in each case. The mean length of procedure was 64 ± 34.5 minutes. A summary of the cases is provided in **Table 1**.

Preprocedure antiplatelet therapy, including aspirin (325 mg) and clopidogrel (75 mg) on a daily basis, was started either on the day of procedure or the night before. Three patients (cases 1, 5, and 7) did not receive any antiplatelet therapy before the procedure owing to the emergent nature of the procedure; they were started on aspirin and clopidogrel postprocedurally. Similarly, 3 patients (cases 9, 10, and 11) received aspirin (325 mg) and prasugrel (10 mg) preoperatively for emergent procedures. A single patient (case 2) received aspirin (325 mg) and Brilinta (180 mg) for preprocedure antiplatelet therapy 13 days after SAH. For all patients in this series, postprocedure antiplatelet therapy consisted of the same regimen as the preprocedure therapy for a period of 3 months, followed by aspirin alone thereafter.

Table 2 shows the ischemic and hemorrhagic events, occlusion rates, and functional outcomes following the deployment of a flow diverter after acute SAH. One patient (case 1) had intraoperative thromboembolic occlusion of the right M3 segment. Similarly, in-stent thrombus was noted during the procedure in 1 patient (case 11), which resolved completely after the administration a bolus of eptifibatide. One patient (case 1) continued to have an extension of SAH and intraparenchymal hemorrhage after the procedure; consequently, this patient did not receive any antiplatelet therapy before or after the procedure. There were no cases of rerupture of the aneurysm. Periprocedural mortality in the first 30 days was 18.2% (2 of 11 cases, cases 1 and 2). The patients in the remaining 9 of 11 cases (81.8%) achieved good functional recovery (Modified Rankin Scale [mRS] scores of 0–2) at the mean clinical follow-up of 23 ± 18.1 months and 100% obliteration of the aneurysm at the mean radiographic follow-up of 24 ± 17.3 months. PED stenosis on follow-up imaging was noted in only 1 case (case 11). Two

Table 1
Summary of our cases of flow diversion after aneurysmal subarachnoid hemorrhage

Case Number	Sex	Age (y)	Hunt and Hess Grade	Time from SAH Presentation to PED (d)	Aneurysm Location	Side	Aneurysms (N)	Morphology/ Shape	Previous Treatment and Type	Procedure	PEDs (N)	Preoperative Antiplatelet Therapy
1	F	63	4	1	ICA: supraclinoid	R	1	Blister	None	PED alone	1	None
2	M	76	4	13[a]	Basilar	NA	1	Dissecting	None	PED alone	1	Aspirin + Brilinta
3	F	57	2	1	VA: V4	L	1	Dissecting	None	PED alone	1	Aspirin + clopidogrel
4	M	54	1	4[b]	ICA: paraophthalmic	L	1	Saccular	None	PED alone	1	Aspirin + clopidogrel
5	M	49	2	1	ICA: SHA	R	1	Saccular	None	PED alone	1	None
6	F	49	5	0	VA: V4	R	1	Blister	None	PED alone	1	Aspirin + clopidogrel
7	F	19	1	0	ICA: paraophthalmic ICA: clinoid	L	2	Blister; blister	None	PED alone	1	None
8	F	50	3	7	ICA: supraclinoid	L	1	Saccular	Yes (coiling)	PED alone	1	Aspirin + clopidogrel
9	F	54	5	0	ICA: paraophthalmic ICA: anterior choroidal PComA	L	3	Saccular; Blister; Saccular	Yes (Coiling); None; None	PED alone[c]	1	Aspirin + prasugrel
10	F	48	1	0	ICA: posterior wall	L	1	Blister	None	PED alone	1	Aspirin + prasugrel
11	F	55	3	0	ICA: paraclinoid	L	1	Fusiform	None	PED and coils	1	Aspirin + prasugrel

Note: some of these cases were previously reported by Lin and colleagues[5] and/or Linfante and colleagues.[6]

Abbreviations: NA, not applicable; PComA, posterior communicating artery; SHA, superior hypophyseal artery.

[a] No aneurysm was seen on angiography on day 0 of presentation. Patient had an extension of the hemorrhage and underwent a second angiogram on day 13, which showed a BA dissecting aneurysm.

[b] Patient was transferred from an outside hospital, and a PED was placed on day 0 after admission.

[c] A single PED was deployed across all 3 aneurysms.

Table 2
Ischemic and hemorrhagic events, occlusion rates, and functional outcomes in our cases after flow diversion

Case Number	TE Comp	Hemorrhagic Comp	Postpro Antiplatelet Therapy	In-PED Stenosis on Follow-up	Imaging Modality Used to Confirm Occlusion	Months After Procedure to Last Imaging Follow-up	Months After Procedure to Last Clinical Follow-up	Aneurysm Obliteration at Last Follow-up	Rerupture	Retreatment	mRS Score On Last Follow-up
1	Distal right M3 thrombus	Yes, sx, (extension of SAH and IPH)	None	NA	NA	NA	NA	NA	NA	NA	6
2	No	No	Aspirin + Brilinta	NA	NA	NA	NA	NA	NA	NA	6
3	No	No	Aspirin + clopidogrel	No	DSA	13	14	Complete	No	No	0
4	No	No	Aspirin + clopidogrel	No	CTA	1	1	Complete	No	No	0
5	No	No	Aspirin + clopidogrel	No	MRA	24	24	Complete	No	No	2
6	No	No	Aspirin + clopidogrel	No	DSA	39	39	Complete	No	No	1
7	No	No	Aspirin + clopidogrel	No	MRA	9	3	Complete	No	No	0
8	No	No	Aspirin + clopidogrel	No	DSA	4	4	Complete	No	No	1
9	No	No	Aspirin + prasugrel	No	MRA	44	44	Complete	No	No	0
10	No	No	Aspirin + prasugrel	No	MRA	37	38	Complete	No	No	0
11	In-PED stenosis	No	Aspirin + prasugrel	Yes	MRA	42	42	Complete	No	No	2

Note: some of these cases were previously reported by Lin and colleagues[5] and/or Linfante and colleagues.[6]

Abbreviations: Comp, complications; CTA, computed tomographic angiography; DSA, digital subtraction angiography; IPH, parenchymal hemorrhage; MRA, magnetic resonance angiography; mRS, Modified Rankin Scale; NA, no follow-up available (patient died); Postpro, postprocedure; sx, symptomatic; TE, thromboembolic.

in a delayed fashion. All 8 patients with blister aneurysms had follow-up digital subtraction angiography, and all had complete occlusion of the aneurysm. Two patients required additional aneurysm treatment: 1 patient with a giant recurrent saccular ICA aneurysm had residual filling of the aneurysm dome 5 months after PED placement and underwent microsurgical bypass and parent vessel sacrifice, and the other patient had a fusiform VA aneurysm that needed a second PED placement 6 months after the initial embolization procedure. One patient had an asymptomatic EVD tract hemorrhage after PED aneurysm treatment. There were no other hemorrhagic complications.

Linfante and colleagues[6] reported 10 cases of ruptured blister aneurysms (8 ICA and 2 MCA) treated with Pipeline flow diversion at 2 institutions. Placement of a single PED resulted in immediate occlusion or near occlusion of the BA in 9 of the 10 patients. In 1 patient, the lesion remained patent and tended to grow despite placement of 3 PEDs in 2 procedures. However, there was no rerupture in this case despite a dual antiplatelet regimen and growth of the lesion. This patient died after the family withdrew care because he had severe vasospasm and poor functional recovery. Among the remaining 9 cases, 8 patients had an mRS score of 0 at 90-day follow-up and 1 had a 90-day mRS score of 1. In the surviving 9 patients, there was complete occlusion of the aneurysm on long-term follow-up angiography.

Hemorrhagic Risk with Dual Antiplatelet Agents After Subarachnoid Hemorrhage

Bodily and colleagues[19] reviewed 17 studies with 212 patients who had dual antiplatelet therapy for stent-assisted coiling in the setting of SAH. Clinically significant intracranial hemorrhagic complications occurred in 8% of patients, including 10% of patients known to have EVDs who had ventricular drain-related hemorrhages. Amenta and colleagues[20] reported 65 patients who underwent stent-assisted coiling in the setting of SAH. There were 15.38% major complications associated with bleeding secondary to antiplatelet therapy and 4.6% of the patients had a fatal hemorrhage. Kung and colleagues[21] reported 131 patients who underwent endovascular treatment with stent-assisted coiling for an acutely ruptured aneurysm as well as ventriculostomy or ventriculoperitoneal shunt placement. The rates of radiographic hemorrhage and symptomatic hemorrhage were 32% and 8% respectively. The risk of hemorrhage after dual antiplatelet use has to be carefully assessed against the risk versus the benefit of aneurysm treatment with other options before choosing flow diversion in patients with aneurysmal SAH.

Blister Aneurysms

Blister aneurysms are uncommon and fragile lesions that commonly occur in the supraclinoid region of the ICA. They have high rates of mortality and morbidity despite multiple treatment strategies and currently there is no optimal treatment option for these lesions. Kalani and colleagues[22] reported 2 cases of blister ICA aneurysms that recurred after clip wrapping. In these cases, the CT angiograms were negative, whereas residual aneurysm was seen on the diagnostic catheter angiogram. They treated both these patients successfully by performing flow diversion on a delayed basis and proposed a strategy of delayed flow diversion after clip wrapping for these aneurysms. Given the success associated with the treatment of these aneurysms with primary flow diversion,[8,15,17] this delayed flow diversion approach may be unnecessary. At our center, these patients are chosen for primary flow diversion.

Risk of Dome Protection and Delayed Flow Diversion After Aneurysmal Rupture

Brinjikji and colleagues[7] reported 31 patients at 2 institutions who were selected for aneurysm dome protection with coils, followed by delayed flow diversion. Four patients could not undergo further flow-diverter therapy: 3 who died as a result of complications of SAH and 1 patient who had permanent morbidity as a result of perioperative ischemic stroke. The median time to treatment was 16 weeks. There were no cases of permanent morbidity or mortality resulting from flow-diverter treatment. The Cerebral Aneurysm Rerupture After Treatment (CARAT) study reported 19 postprocedural ruptures in 1001 patients treated with coil embolization or surgical clipping of ruptured intracranial aneurysms.[23] Median time to rerupture was 3 days, and rerupture led to death in 58% of the patients. The degree of aneurysm occlusion after treatment was strongly associated with the risk of rerupture (17.6% for <70% aneurysm occlusion). In the setting of rupture, our goal is primarily to protect the dome of the aneurysm and obliterate high-risk regions like daughter sacs or focal outpouchings. A balance should be maintained between achieving packing density with coils that is sufficient to secure the aneurysm and avoiding aneurysm rupture or parent vessel compromise caused by excessive packing. Given the risk of immediate and late rebleeding, we perform a diagnostic angiogram on all our patients before discharge to check aneurysm occlusion and perform flow diversion if needed before discharge.

Flow Diversion Is Associated with Better Long-term Aneurysm Occlusion Rates

Flow diversion is intended for endoluminal reconstruction of the parent vessel compared with traditional endosaccular aneurysm treatments. A recent pooled analysis of the International Retrospective Study of Pipeline Embolization Device (IntrePED), Pipeline for Uncoilable or Failed Aneurysms (PUFS) trial, and the Aneurysm Study of Pipeline in an Observational Registry (ASPIRe), included 1221 aneurysms and reported complete aneurysm occlusion rates of 85.5% at 1 year.[24] This rate is twice the occlusion rate of simple coiling for all aneurysms, despite patients with complex aneurysms being treated by flow diversion and these patients being expected to have poorer occlusion rates compared with all coiled aneurysms. At our institute, we use flow diversion in the acute rupture setting only for good-grade patients (Hunt & Hess grades 1–3) who have an aneurysm that cannot be safely dome protected by traditional endovascular or microsurgical means because only the use of dual antiplatelet therapy in the ruptured setting would be justified in these patients.

Coiling-assisted Flow Diversion

Adjunctive coiling during flow diversion has been proposed to ensure adequate aneurysm thrombosis in a quick manner if feasible, especially in ruptured aneurysms. The delayed occlusion rates after flow diversion with coiling versus flow diversion alone have been shown to be better.[25] The coils also serve as a conduit to support the PED in giant fusiform aneurysms in which a long length of the parent artery is aneurysmal. In these cases, the potential drawbacks of coiling are perforator occlusions, accelerated thrombosis leading to aneurysm rupture, and difficulty in visualizing the PED when there are coils in the aneurysm sac. The IntrePED showed that coiling in conjunction with PED treatment required a significantly longer procedure (135.8 vs 96.7 minutes; $P<.0001$) and resulted in higher neurologic morbidity (12.5% vs 7.8%; $P = .13$).[26] Adjunctive coiling with flow diversion may be best reserved for patients with a clear history of rupture or sentinel headaches or to support the PED in patients with giant fusiform aneurysms. In such cases, the coiling catheter is typically jailed, and 1.5 loops of the coil are deployed in the aneurysm before the PED is deployed. The goal is to achieve loose packing to avoid perforator occlusion and accelerated thrombosis.[5]

SHIELD TECHNOLOGY MAY INCREASE THE SAFETY OF FLOW DIVERSION IN ANEURYSMAL SUBARACHNOID HEMORRHAGE

The PED with Shield Technology (PED + Shield, Medtronic) is a phosphorylcholine surface modification of the PED flow diverter that has shown reduction in material thrombogenicity in vitro and in an ex vivo arteriovenous shunt model in a nonhuman primate.[27] It is currently approved for clinical use in Australia but not in the United States. Anecdotal reports (Haggstrom K, personal communication from Medtronic, 2017) suggest that the Australian centers that have the largest human experience with this technology use dual antiplatelet therapy after treatment with a PED + Shield only for 1 month and have recently published their use of this device using aspirin as the sole oral antiplatelet therapy and a single intravenous loading dose of abciximab in the setting of aneurysm rupture.[28] Further development of this technology may allow flow diversion with a single antiplatelet agent, and thus may broaden the use of flow diversion in this setting.

SUMMARY

Flow diversion is not the primary treatment of choice after aneurysmal SAH but is a reasonable last option if other, safer options are not available to treat the aneurysm. In the setting of acute aneurysm rupture, protection of the aneurysm dome followed by delayed flow diversion is a safer choice than primary flow diversion. Our experience and review of the literature show the feasibility of flow diversion after aneurysmal SAH as primary treatment or in a subacute fashion after dome protection.

Careful patient selection, selective use of coiling, timing of flow diversion after dome protection, and timing of heparin and antiplatelet therapy in the periprocedural period improve the safety of flow diversion as a strategy to achieve permanent aneurysm occlusion in the rupture setting. Shield technology may decrease the duration of, or need for, dual antiplatelet therapy, thereby making flow diversion safer in the rupture setting.

DISCLOSURE

Dr E.I. Levy has shareholder/ownership interests in Intratech Medical Ltd, Blockade Medical LLC, and NeXtGen Biologics. He serves as a national principal investigator for the Covidien US SWIFT PRIME trials and receives honoraria for training and lecturing from that company. He receives compensation from Abbott for carotid training sessions for physicians. He serves as a consultant to Pulsar and Blockade Medical and on the Acute Ischemic Stroke Clinical Advisory Board for Stryker and the Advisory Board for NeXtGen Biologics and MEDX. Dr A.H. Siddiqui has financial interests in Buffalo Technology Partners Inc, Cardinal, International Medical Distribution Partners, Medina Medical Systems, Neuro Technology Investors, StimSox, and Valor Medical. He serves as a consultant to Amnis Therapeutics Ltd, Cerebrotech Medical Systems Inc, CereVasc LLC, Codman, Corindus Inc, Covidien (acquired by Medtronic), GuidePoint Global Consulting, Lazarus (acquired by Medtronic), Medina Medical (acquired by Medtronic), Medtronic, MicroVention, Neuravi, Penumbra, Pulsar Vascular, Rapid Medical, Rebound Medical, Reverse Medical (acquired by Medtronic), Silk Road Medical Inc, Stryker, The Stroke Project Inc, Three Rivers Medical Inc, and W.L. Gore & Associates. He is a principal investigator or serves on the National Steering Committee for the following trials: Covidien SWIFT PRIME, LARGE, Medtronic SWIFT DIRECT, MicroVention CONFIDENCE, MicroVention FRED, Penumbra 3D Separator, Penumbra COMPASS, Penumbra INVEST, and POSITIVE Trial. He is a member of the board of the Intersocietal Accreditation Committee. Dr K.V. Snyder serves on the speakers' bureaus of Toshiba and the Jacobs Institute. Drs S.K. Natarajan, H. Shallwani, V.S. Fennell, J.S. Beecher, H.J. Shakir, and J.M. Davies have nothing to disclose.

REFERENCES

1. Molyneux A, Kerr R, Stratton I, et al. International Subarachnoid Aneurysm Trial (ISAT) of neurosurgical clipping versus endovascular coiling in 2143 patients with ruptured intracranial aneurysms: a randomised trial. Lancet 2002;360(9342):1267–74.

2. Molyneux AJ, Birks J, Clarke A, et al. The durability of endovascular coiling versus neurosurgical clipping of ruptured cerebral aneurysms: 18 year follow-up of the UK cohort of the International Subarachnoid Aneurysm Trial (ISAT). Lancet 2015; 385(9969):691–7.

3. Molyneux AJ, Kerr RS, Yu LM, et al. International Subarachnoid Aneurysm Trial (ISAT) of neurosurgical clipping versus endovascular coiling in 2143 patients with ruptured intracranial aneurysms: a randomised comparison of effects on survival, dependency, seizures, rebleeding, subgroups, and aneurysm occlusion. Lancet 2005;366(9488): 809–17.

4. Chalouhi N, Tjoumakaris S, Starke RM, et al. Comparison of flow diversion and coiling in large unruptured intracranial saccular aneurysms. Stroke 2013; 44(8):2150–4.

5. Lin N, Brouillard AM, Keigher KM, et al. Utilization of Pipeline embolization device for treatment of ruptured intracranial aneurysms: US multicenter experience. J Neurointerv Surg 2015;7(11):808–15.

6. Linfante I, Mayich M, Sonig A, et al. Flow diversion with Pipeline Embolic Device as treatment of subarachnoid hemorrhage secondary to blister aneurysms: dual-center experience and review of the literature. J Neurointerv Surg 2017;9(1):29–33.

7. Brinjikji W, Piano M, Fang S, et al. Treatment of ruptured complex and large/giant ruptured cerebral aneurysms by acute coiling followed by staged flow diversion. J Neurosurg 2016;125(1):120–7.

8. Chalouhi N, Zanaty M, Tjoumakaris S, et al. Treatment of blister-like aneurysms with the Pipeline embolization device. Neurosurgery 2014;74(5): 527–32 [discussion: 532].

9. Chalouhi N, Zanaty M, Whiting A, et al. Treatment of ruptured intracranial aneurysms with the Pipeline embolization device. Neurosurgery 2015;76(2): 165–72 [discussion: 172].

10. Chan RS, Mak CH, Wong AK, et al. Use of the Pipeline embolization device to treat recently ruptured dissecting cerebral aneurysms. Interv Neuroradiol 2014;20(4):436–41.

11. Cinar C, Oran I, Bozkaya H, et al. Endovascular treatment of ruptured blister-like aneurysms with special reference to the flow-diverting strategy. Neuroradiology 2013;55(4):441–7.

12. Cruz JP, O'Kelly C, Kelly M, et al. Pipeline Embolization Device in aneurysmal subarachnoid hemorrhage. AJNR Am J Neuroradiol 2013;34(2):271–6.

13. de Barros Faria M, Castro RN, Lundquist J, et al. The role of the Pipeline Embolization Device for the treatment of dissecting intracranial aneurysms. AJNR Am J Neuroradiol 2011;32(11):2192–5.

14. McAuliffe W, Wenderoth JD. Immediate and midterm results following treatment of recently ruptured intracranial aneurysms with the Pipeline Embolization Device. AJNR Am J Neuroradiol 2012;33(3):487–93.

15. Yoon JW, Siddiqui AH, Dumont TM, et al. For the Endovascular Neurosurgery Research Group. Feasibility and safety of Pipeline Embolization Device in patients with ruptured carotid blister aneurysms. Neurosurgery 2014;75(4):419–29 [discussion: 429].

16. Martin AR, Cruz JP, Matouk CC, et al. The Pipeline flow-diverting stent for exclusion of ruptured intracranial aneurysms with difficult morphologies. Neurosurgery 2012;70(1 Suppl Operative):21–8 [discussion: 28].

17. Consoli A, Nappini S, Renieri L, et al. Treatment of two blood blister-like aneurysms with flow diverter stenting. J Neurointerv Surg 2012;4(3):e4.

18. Nerva JD, Morton RP, Levitt MR, et al. Pipeline Embolization Device as primary treatment for blister aneurysms and iatrogenic pseudoaneurysms of the internal carotid artery. J Neurointerv Surg 2015; 7(3):210–6.

19. Bodily KD, Cloft HJ, Lanzino G, et al. Stent-assisted coiling in acutely ruptured intracranial aneurysms: a qualitative, systematic review of the literature. AJNR Am J Neuroradiol 2011;32(7):1232–6.

20. Amenta PS, Dalyai RT, Kung D, et al. Stent-assisted coiling of wide-necked aneurysms in the setting of acute subarachnoid hemorrhage: experience in 65 patients. Neurosurgery 2012;70(6):1415–29 [discussion: 1429].

21. Kung DK, Policeni BA, Capuano AW, et al. Risk of ventriculostomy-related hemorrhage in patients with acutely ruptured aneurysms treated using stent-assisted coiling. J Neurosurg 2011;114(4):1021–7.

22. Kalani MY, Albuquerque FC, Levitt M, et al. Pipeline embolization for definitive endoluminal reconstruction of blister-type carotid aneurysms after clip wrapping. J Neurointerv Surg 2016;8(5):495–500.

23. Johnston SC, Dowd CF, Higashida RT, et al. Predictors of rehemorrhage after treatment of ruptured intracranial aneurysms: the Cerebral Aneurysm Rerupture After Treatment (CARAT) study. Stroke 2008;39(1):120–5.

24. Kallmes DF, Brinjikji W, Cekirge S, et al. Safety and efficacy of the Pipeline Embolization Device for treatment of intracranial aneurysms: a pooled analysis of 3 large studies. J Neurosurg 2016;1–6.

25. Park MS, Nanaszko M, Sanborn MR, et al. Re-treatment rates after treatment with the Pipeline Embolization Device alone versus Pipeline and coil embolization of cerebral aneurysms: a single-center experience. J Neurosurg 2016;125(1):137–44.

26. Park MS, Kilburg C, Taussky P, et al. Pipeline Embolization Device with or without adjunctive coil embolization: analysis of complications from the IntrePED Registry. AJNR Am J Neuroradiol 2016;37(6):1127–31.

27. Hagen MW, Girdhar G, Wainwright J, et al. Thrombogenicity of flow diverters in an ex vivo shunt model: effect of phosphorylcholine surface modification. J Neurointerv Surg 2016. [Epub ahead of print].

28. Chiu A, Ramesh R, Wenderoth J, et al. Use of aspirin as sole oral antiplatelet therapy in acute flow diversion for ruptured dissecting aneurysm. J Neurointerv Surg 2016. [Epub ahead of print].

Management of Small Incidental Intracranial Aneurysms

Jan-Karl Burkhardt, MD, Arnau Benet, MD,
Michael T. Lawton, MD*

KEYWORDS

- Unruptured intracranial aneurysms (UIA) • Small-sized UIAs • Incidental aneurysm
- Microsurgical clipping • Endovascular coiling

KEY POINTS

- The decision-making process for treatment of small intracranial aneurysms (UIAs) is based on aneurysm rupture risk factors and needs to be weighed against the complication risk during aneurysm treatment.
- Scores to calculate the individual rupture risk in patients with unruptured intracranial aneurysms are helpful during the decision-making process.
- Microsurgical or endovascular aneurysm treatment is recommended for small UIAs in a high-volume neurosurgical center with a low complication risk.

INTRODUCTION

Advances in neuroimaging and its widespread use for screening have increased diagnosis rate of unruptured intracranial aneurysms (UIAs), including small-sized UIAs[1,2] (**Figs. 1–3**). This growing rate of patients presenting with small, incidental UIAs raise the question whether treatment is needed. Although the estimated 3% prevalence of intracranial aneurysms is low, aneurysm rupture causing subarachnoid hemorrhage (SAH) can be devastating, with morbidity and mortality rates around 25% and 40%, respectively.[3] Patients presenting with ruptured aneurysms need to be treated because they are at high risk for rerupture within the first days and weeks.[1] Both microsurgical clipping as well as endovascular coiling are the current treatment options of choice for ruptured or unruptured aneurysms.[1,2,4,5] Clinical management of patients with UIAs requires a fine judgment of the risk of aneurysm rupture and

a decision to observe, versus the risk of complications from surgical or endovascular treatment and a decision to intervene, which is patient specific. Rupture risk ranges between 0.1% and 4% per year and depends on different risk factors,[6,7] such as aneurysm size and location. Aneurysm size is one of the most important factors in assessing rupture risk in UIAs. Patients with larger aneurysms have a higher risk of aneurysm rupture. The International Study of Unruptured Intracranial Aneurysms (ISUIA) trial and the Unruptured Cerebral Aneurysm Study (UCAS) stratified the risk of rupture for UIAs according to aneurysm size, which showed a small annual rupture risk for UIAs less than 7 mm.[8,9] This review discusses the current evidence for the management of small UIAs.

PATIENT EVALUATION OVERVIEW

There are several modifiable and nonmodifiable patient risk factors for small UIA rupture, which

Department of Neurological Surgery, University of California San Francisco, San Francisco, CA, USA
* Corresponding author. Department of Neurological Surgery, University of California San Francisco, 400 Parnassus Avenue, San Francisco, CA 94143.
E-mail address: Michael.Lawton@ucsf.edu

Neurosurg Clin N Am 28 (2017) 389–396
http://dx.doi.org/10.1016/j.nec.2017.02.006
1042-3680/17/© 2017 Elsevier Inc. All rights reserved.

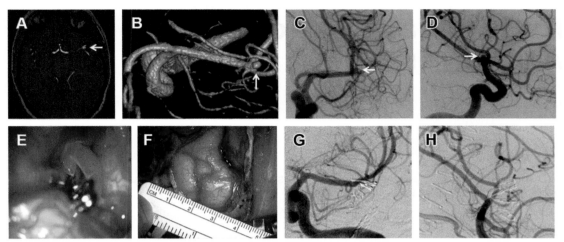

Fig. 1. This 39-year-old woman was diagnosed during migraine workup with an incidental unruptured middle cerebral artery (MCA) bifurcation aneurysm (*A*, MRI/magnetic resonance angiography [MRA] axial time-of-flight MRA). Catheter angiography confirmed the small UIA with a maximal size of 2.4 mm on lateral (*D*), anteroposterior (*C*), and 3-dimentional reconstruction (*B*) Arrow indicates aneurysm. The patient had a PHASES score of 3 (1 point for hypertension and 2 points for MCA location), with an individual 5-year risk of aneurysm rupture of 0.7%. Given her young age and a life expectancy of greater than 50 years (cumulative rupture risk within 50 years of 7%), she preferred aneurysm treatment. The aneurysm was microsurgically clipped through a mini pterional craniotomy (*E, F*). Postoperative catheter angiography confirmed complete clipping without remnant (*G, H*).

must be taken into account during decision-making (**Table 1**). These factors influence the treating physician to recommend aneurysm treatment or clinical follow-up with or without medical treatment. In general, patients with small but symptomatic UIAs should be treated to prevent neurologic deficit progression or persistence. An example of such a case would be a posterior communicating artery (PCoA) aneurysm causing oculomotor nerve palsy due to compression or irritation of the nerve, without aneurysm rupture. Younger patients will benefit from aneurysm surgery, because the cumulative risk of rupture leads to a higher rupture risk than the aneurysm

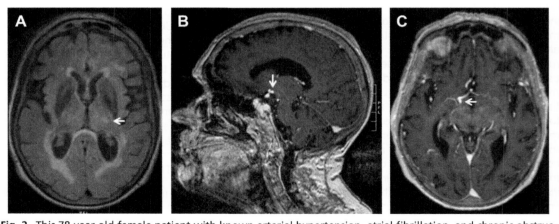

Fig. 2. This 78-year-old female patient with known arterial hypertension, atrial fibrillation, and chronic obstructive pulmonary disease was diagnosed with a left thalamic stroke and right-sided paresis. During stroke workup, a right-sided unruptured, incidental internal carotid artery (ICA) terminus aneurysm was diagnosed. (*A*) Axial MRI showed the thalamic stroke as well as her small vessel disease Arrow indicates thalamic stroke. (*B, C*) MRI showed the 4-mm ICA terminus aneurysms (axial and sagittal T1-weighted images with contrast) Arrow indicates aneurysm. Giving her age, the stroke, as well as the small aneurysm size, clinical and radiological follow-up was favored over aneurysm treatment with a high complication risk profile. Her PHASES score was 3 (1 point each for age, hypertension, and aneurysm location) with an individual 5-year risk of aneurysm rupture of 0.7%.

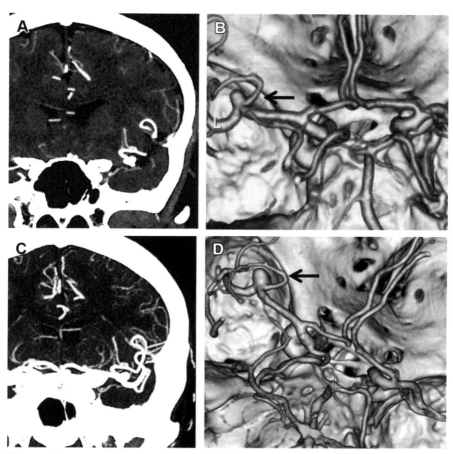

Fig. 3. This 67-year-old woman was diagnosed with an unruptured incidental left MCA bifurcation aneurysm after she had a fall and hit her head. With a size of approximately 4.5 mm and a PHASES score of 2 (2 points for aneurysm location), clinical and radiological follow-up was favored with an individual 5-year risk of aneurysm rupture of only 0.4%. At the 1-year follow-up, CTA aneurysm size was stable (*A, B*). Three years later, the aneurysm increased in size to approximately 6 mm (*C, D*) Arrow indicates aneurysm. Treatment was indicated because of the aneurysm growth, and microsurgical clipping was favored over endovascular coiling because of the wide aneurysm neck and aneurysm location.

treatment complication risk. Also, other instances whereby the treatment risk is lower than the rupture risk include a history of SAH from another ruptured aneurysm, aneurysmal family history in first-degree relatives, and an underlying genetic disease, including polycystic kidney disease or Marfan syndrome. Aneurysm characteristics, such as anatomic location, a borderline size of 5 to 7 mm, and aneurysm shape (such as blebs or multi-lobulated aneurysms), are factors that favor treatment. Useful tools to calculate the individual aneurysm rupture risk are the PHASES score (**Table 2**) and the UIA treatment score (**Table 3**), which can be used to compare with the possible complication rate during aneurysm treatment (**Fig. 1**).[6,7] Another risk factor score for UIA proposed by Chalouhi and colleagues[10]

includes type A factors that favor intervention over observation and type B factors that warrant a strong consideration for treatment independent of size. Type A factors include active smoking, arterial hypertension, posterior circulation aneurysm, prior SAH, familial SAH, and/or aspect ratio greater than 3. Type B factors include young patient age, change in size or configuration of aneurysm, presence of multiple aneurysms, multilobed configuration, or symptomatic aneurysm (emboli or mass effect). In patients with unruptured aneurysm measuring 5 to 7 mm, treatment is recommended if any risk factor (A or B) is present, whereas patients with unruptured aneurysms less than 5 mm should only be treated in the presence of 2 or more type A or any type B risk factors.[10]

Table 1
Summary of modifiable and nonmodifiable factors influencing decision-making process in small unruptured intracranial aneurysms

Nonmodifiable Factors	In Favor of Aneurysm Treatment	In Favor of Clinical Follow-up
Patient age (y)	<50	>70
Ethnic background	—	Japanese, Finnish
Genetic diseases	Polycystic kidney disease, Marfan syndrome	—
Family history	Two first-degree relatives	Second- or third-degree relatives
Previous SAH	Generally recommended	—
Aneurysm characteristics		
Size	5–7 mm	—
Location	Posterior circulation, MCA, ACoA	<5 mm
Blebs/multi-lobulated	Generally recommended	ICA (cavernous sinus)
Modifiable Factors to be Treated with or Without Aneurysm Treatment		
Hypertension Nicotine abuse Diabetes mellitus Alcohol consumption Hyperlipidemia		

Abbreviations: ACoA, anterior communicating artery; ICA, internal carotid artery; MCA, middle cerebral artery.

When a decision has been made to manage a small aneurysm conservatively, follow-up imaging is typically recommended at yearly intervals to monitor for enlargement (**Fig. 2**). A growing aneurysm, even if it remains less than 7 mm in diameter, is one that should be strongly considered for treatment and the initial management decision reversed (**Fig. 3**). These dynamic aneurysms suggest that structural weaknesses in the aneurysm wall or more malignant hemodynamics are at play and that the associated risk of rupture exceeds that predicted by size alone.

MEDICAL TREATMENT OPTIONS

Modifiable risk factors for aneurysm rupture include hypertension, diabetes mellitus, hyperlipidemia, nicotine abuse, and alcohol consumption. These risk factors should all be treated, even if the aneurysm itself is not subject to treatment. Cessation of smoking and reduction of alcohol intake is recommended in general for all patients with aneurysms to prevent aneurysm growth.[11] Hypertension should be medically treated to normal pressure range to prevent rupture risk as recommended in other vascular diseases.[12] Also it has been described that hypertension may lead to the formation of intracranial aneurysms and growth.[11,13] Because there are no specific guidelines for antihypertensive medication specific to UIAs, general guidelines for the treatment of hypertension should

be followed.[14] Diabetes mellitus type 2 is also a known vascular risk factor; therefore, it should be treated when diagnosed in patients with UIAs. Although there is controversy in the literature regarding hypercholesterolemia, hyperlipidemia, and aneurysm rupture risk, patients should be medically treated and their blood levels of these agents controlled with statin drugs.[15]

SURGICAL TREATMENT OPTIONS

Microsurgical clipping and endovascular coiling are the gold standards for the occlusion of unruptured saccular aneurysms.[5,16] Small unruptured fusiform aneurysms are best treated with surgical trapping plus bypass or endovascular flow diverter devices depending on aneurysm location.[17]

For there to be a benefit from treatment, the complication risk of these procedures must be lower than the rupture risk of the untreated aneurysm, which is low in small unruptured aneurysms. Treatment should be only recommended in high-volume centers and by expert surgeons with a high caseload and a low morbidity rate. It has been shown that the morbidity and mortality rate of both endovascular and surgical treatment groups regarding unruptured aneurysms is significantly lower in patients treated in high-volume centers.[18–20] However, these studies did not differentiate between aneurysm sizes of the treated unruptured aneurysms.

Table 2
The PHASES aneurysm risk score

PHASES Aneurysm Risk Score		Points
(P) Population	North American, European (other than Finnish)	0
	Japanese	3
	Finnish	5
(H) Hypertension	No	0
	Yes	1
(A) Age	<70 y	0
	≥70 y	1
(S) Size of aneurysm	<7.0 mm	0
	7.0–9.9 mm	3
	10.0–19.9 mm	6
	≥20 mm	10
(E) Earlier SAH from another aneurysm	No	0
	Yes	1
(S) Site of aneurysm	ICA	0
	MCA	2
	ACA/Pcom/posterior	4

PHASES Risk Score	5-y Risk of Aneurysm Rupture Rate
<2	0.4% (0.1–1.5)
3	0.7% (0.2–1.5)
4	0.9% (0.3–2.0)
5	1.3% (0.8–2.4)
6	1.7% (1.1–2.7)
7	2.4% (1.6–3.3)
8	3.2% (2.3–4.4)
9	4.3% (2.9–6.1)
10	5.3% (3.5–8)
11	7.2% (5–10.2)
>12	17.8% (15.2–20.7)

The number of points associated with each indicator can be added up to obtain the total risk score.

Abbreviations: ACA, anterior cerebral arteries (including the anterior cerebral artery, anterior communicating artery, and pericallosal artery); ICA, internal carotid artery; MCA, middle cerebral artery; Pcom, posterior communicating artery; posterior, posterior circulation (including the vertebral artery, basilar artery, cerebellar arteries, and posterior cerebral artery).

From Greving JP, Wermer MJ, Brown RD Jr, et al. Development of the PHASES score for prediction of risk of rupture of intracranial aneurysms: a pooled analysis of six prospective cohort studies. Lancet Neurol. 2014;13(1):64.

Microsurgical clipping for small UIAs is effective and should be considered as first-line treatment because of its durability, with lower recurrence rate and retreatment rate compared with endovascular coiling.[21–24] This recommendation applies especially to younger patients with a long life expectancy. Also patients with small aneurysms commonly have wide aneurysm necks, which are more favorable for surgical clipping than endovascular coiling.[24,25] In older patients with a higher risk profile for open surgery, endovascular coiling might be preferable. However, in such a situation, it is questionable if the treatment complication risk in older patients outweighs the rupture risk for small UIAs.

EVALUATION OF OUTCOME AND LONG-TERM RECOMMENDATIONS

Because patients with UIAs are asymptomatic at initial presentation, clinical outcome is measured by any neurologic impairment after treatment. Both microsurgical clipping and endovascular coiling have certain risk profiles for patients depending on its localization and patient morbidity risk factors.[18–20]

Radiological outcome is measured by complete aneurysm occlusion on postoperative angiography. The catheter angiography remains the imaging modality of choice to detect small aneurysm remnants, but it carries the risk of catheter-associated

Table 3
The unruptured intracranial aneurysm treatment score

Categories	Favors UIA Repair	Favors UIA Conservative Treatment
Age (single) (y)		
<40	4	—
40–60	3	—
61–70	2	—
71–80	1	—
>80	0	—
Risk factor incidence (multiple)		
Previous SAH from a different aneurysm	4	—
Familial intracranial aneurysm or SAH	3	—
Japanese, Finish, Inuit ethnicity	2	—
Current cigarette smoking	3	—
Hypertension (systolic BP >140 mm HG)	2	—
Autosomal-polycystic kidney disease	2	—
Current drug abuse (cocaine, amphetamine)	2	—
Current alcohol abuse	1	—
Clinical symptoms related to UIA (multiple)		
Cranial nerve deficit	4	—
Clinical or radiological mass effect	4	—
Thromboembolic events from the aneurysm	3	—
Epilepsy	1	—
Other (multiple)		
Reduced quality of life due to fear or rupture	2	—
Aneurysm multiplicity	1	—
Life expectancy due to chronic and/or malignant diseases (single) (y)		
<5	—	4
5–10	—	3
>10	—	2
Comorbid disease (multiple)		
Neurocognitive disorder	—	3
Coagulopathies, thrombophilic diseases	—	2
Psychiatric disorders	—	2
Maximum diameter (single)		
<3.9 mm	0	—
4.0–6.9 mm	1	—
7.0–12.9 mm	2	—
13.0–24.9 mm	3	—
>25 mm	4	—
Morphology (multiple)		
Irregularity or lobulation	3	—
Size ratio >3 or aspect ratio >1.6	1	—
Location (single)		
BasA bifurcation	5	—
Vertebral/basilar artery	4	—
AcomA or PcomA	2	—

(continued on next page)

Table 3
(continued)

Categories	Favors UIA Repair	Favors UIA Conservative Treatment
Other (multiple)		
Aneurysm growth on serial imaging	4	—
Aneurysm de novo formation on serial imaging	3	—
Contralateral steno-occlusive vessel disease	1	—
Age-related risk (single) (y)		
<40	—	0
41–60	—	1
61–70	—	3
71–80	—	4
>80	—	5
Aneurysm size-related risk (single) (mm)		
<6.0	—	0
6.0–10.0	—	1
10.1–20.0	—	3
>20	—	5
Aneurysm complexity-related risk		
High	—	3
Low	—	0
Intervention-related risk constant	—	5

To calculate a management recommendation for a UIA, the number of points corresponding to each patient- (white), aneurysm- (light gray), or treatment-related (dark gray) feature are added up for both "in favor of UIA repair" and "in favor of UIA conservative management." For cases with a score difference of 3 or more points UIA repair or conservative management are recommended; for cases with a score difference of ±2 points or less, the recommendation is "not definitive" and additional factors apart from those used in this score may be considered for final decision making.

Abbreviations: AComA, anterior communicating artery; BasA, basilar artery; BP, blood pressure; multiple, multiple selection category; PComA, posterior communicating artery; single, single selection category.

From Etminan N, Brown RD Jr, Beseoglu K, et al. The unruptured intracranial aneurysm treatment score: a multidisciplinary consensus. Neurology 2015;85:884; with permission.

stroke. Computed tomography angiography can be used as an alternative imaging modality but has a lower sensitivity to detect small aneurysm remnants compared with the catheter angiography.[26]

Long-term radiological follow-up is recommended even in patients without any neurologic deficits to exclude aneurysm reoccurrence or development of a de novo aneurysm. The authors recommend a catheter angiography in 3 to 5 years, similar to previously published studies.[22]

SUMMARY/DISCUSSION

The clinical management of patients with small-sized UIAs is based on aneurysm rupture prevention, which depends on both fixed and variable risk factors. Treatment of small UIAs requires fine judgment of the risk of aneurysm rupture versus the risk of treatment complications. Experienced cerebrovascular teams recommend treating UIAs in young patients or in patients with more than

one aneurysm rupture risk factor who also have a reasonable life expectancy. However, individual overall assessment of risk is critical for patients with UIAs to decide the next steps of care. Aneurysm rupture risk scores, which estimate the risk of aneurysm rupture based on patient-specific risk factors, are useful tools to assist decision-making.

REFERENCES

1. Fusco MR, Ogilvy CS. Surgical and endovascular management of cerebral aneurysms. Int Anesthesiol Clin 2015;53:146–65.
2. Wiebers DO, Whisnant JP, Huston J 3rd, et al. Unruptured intracranial aneurysms: natural history, clinical outcome, and risks of surgical and endovascular treatment. Lancet 2003;362:103–10.
3. Vlak MH, Algra A, Brandenburg R, et al. Prevalence of unruptured intracranial aneurysms, with emphasis on sex, age, comorbidity, country, and time period: a

systematic review and meta-analysis. Lancet Neurol 2011;10:626–36.

4. Spetzler RF, McDougall CG, Zabramski JM, et al. The barrow ruptured aneurysm trial: 6-year results. J Neurosurg 2015;123:609–17.

5. Bekelis K, Gottlieb DJ, Su Y, et al. Comparison of clipping and coiling in elderly patients with unruptured cerebral aneurysms. J Neurosurg 2017; 126(3):811–8.

6. Backes D, Vergouwen MD, Tiel Groenestege AT, et al. PHASES score for prediction of intracranial aneurysm growth. Stroke 2015;46:1221–6.

7. Etminan N, Brown RD Jr, Beseoglu K, et al. The unruptured intracranial aneurysm treatment score: a multidisciplinary consensus. Neurology 2015;85: 881–9.

8. Unruptured intracranial aneurysms–risk of rupture and risks of surgical intervention. International Study of Unruptured Intracranial Aneurysms Investigators. N Engl J Med 1998;339:1725–33.

9. Investigators UJ, Morita A, Kirino T, et al. The natural course of unruptured cerebral aneurysms in a Japanese cohort. N Engl J Med 2012;366:2474–82.

10. Chalouhi N, Dumont AS, Randazzo C, et al. Management of incidentally discovered intracranial vascular abnormalities. Neurosurg Focus 2011;31:E1.

11. Etminan N, Beseoglu K, Steiger HJ, et al. The impact of hypertension and nicotine on the size of ruptured intracranial aneurysms. J Neurol Neurosurg Psychiatr 2011;82:4–7.

12. Rapsomaniki E, Timmis A, George J, et al. Blood pressure and incidence of twelve cardiovascular diseases: lifetime risks, healthy life-years lost, and age-specific associations in 1.25 million people. Lancet 2014;383:1899–911.

13. Lindgren AE, Kurki MI, Riihinen A, et al. Hypertension predisposes to the formation of saccular intracranial aneurysms in 467 unruptured and 1053 ruptured patients in Eastern Finland. Ann Med 2014;46:169–76.

14. Mankin LA. Update in hypertension therapy. Med Clin North Am 2016;100:665–93.

15. Lindgren AE, Kurki MI, Riihinen A, et al. Type 2 diabetes and risk of rupture of saccular intracranial aneurysm in eastern Finland. Diabetes Care 2013; 36:2020–6.

16. Ajiboye N, Chalouhi N, Starke RM, et al. Unruptured cerebral aneurysms: evaluation and management. ScientificWorldJournal 2015;2015:954954.

17. Sanai N, Zador Z, Lawton MT. Bypass surgery for complex brain aneurysms: an assessment of intracranial-intracranial bypass. Neurosurgery 2009;65:670–83 [discussion: 83].

18. Barker FG 2nd, Amin-Hanjani S, Butler WE, et al. In-hospital mortality and morbidity after surgical treatment of unruptured intracranial aneurysms in the United States, 1996-2000: the effect of hospital and surgeon volume. Neurosurgery 2003;52:995–1007 [discussion: 9].

19. Hoh BL, Rabinov JD, Pryor JC, et al. In-hospital morbidity and mortality after endovascular treatment of unruptured intracranial aneurysms in the United States, 1996-2000: effect of hospital and physician volume. AJNR Am J Neuroradiol 2003;24:1409–20.

20. Brinjikji W, Rabinstein AA, Lanzino G, et al. Patient outcomes are better for unruptured cerebral aneurysms treated at centers that preferentially treat with endovascular coiling: a study of the national inpatient sample 2001-2007. AJNR Am J Neuroradiol 2011;32:1065–70.

21. David CA, Vishteh AG, Spetzler RF, et al. Late angiographic follow-up review of surgically treated aneurysms. J Neurosurg 1999;91:396–401.

22. Brown MA, Parish J, Guandique CF, et al. A long-term study of durability and risk factors for aneurysm recurrence after microsurgical clip ligation. J Neurosurg 2017;126(3):819–24.

23. Chalouhi N, Bovenzi CD, Thakkar V, et al. Long-term catheter angiography after aneurysm coil therapy: results of 209 patients and predictors of delayed recurrence and retreatment. J Neurosurg 2014; 121:1102–6.

24. Davies JM, Lawton MT. Advances in open microsurgery for cerebral aneurysms. Neurosurgery 2014; 74(Suppl 1):S7–16.

25. Nasr DM, Brown RD Jr. Management of unruptured intracranial aneurysms. Curr Cardiol Rep 2016;18:86.

26. Lu L, Zhang LJ, Poon CS, et al. Digital subtraction CT angiography for detection of intracranial aneurysms: comparison with three-dimensional digital subtraction angiography. Radiology 2012;262:605–12.

Surgical Management of Incidental Gliomas

Imran Noorani, MB BChir, MRCS[a,b], Nader Sanai, MD[a,*]

KEYWORDS

- Incidental gliomas • Symptomatic gliomas • Low-grade gliomas • Intrinsic brain tumors

KEY POINTS

- Detailed imaging studies of the brain help to discover gliomas incidentally before the onset of any clinical symptoms or signs.
- These tumors represent early stage gliomas; left untreated, they are likely to become symptomatic and transform to malignant gliomas, with their associated aggressive features.
- A greater extent of resection of low-grade gliomas has been shown to delay the onset of malignant transformation and prolong patient survival.
- Incidental gliomas are smaller and less likely to be in eloquent brain locations than symptomatic gliomas.

INTRODUCTION

Low-grade gliomas (LGG; World Health Organization grade II) are a heterogeneous population of intrinsic brain tumors whose natural history is to evolve to higher grade tumors. Over the last few decades, significant advances in the management of LGGs have been made, particularly in the areas of neuroimaging, treatment paradigms, and the genetic make-up of these tumors. However, important questions remain to be answered. One aspect that has been explored more recently is the management of LGG that present incidentally without any obvious clinical signs when they are investigated with an MRI study for unrelated symptoms, such as headache or dizziness. These incidental gliomas are relatively rare and we are only beginning to understand their clinical and biological features. In this review, we discuss the characteristics of incidental gliomas, and their management, with a particular emphasis on their surgical treatment.

LGG constitute 15% of all adult brain tumors, and they most commonly present with seizures (in 80% of cases).[1] A model for the natural history of gliomas posits 4 phases: (1) the occult stage, in which tumor-initiating cells proliferate but there is no detectable tumor on MRI; (2) the clinically silent stage, in which tumor mass becomes apparent on MRI but the patient does not have any symptoms (incidental glioma); (3) the symptomatic stage, in which the tumor elicits symptoms such as seizures or weakness; and (4) malignant transformation, in which the LGG switches to a more biologically aggressive high-grade glioma.[2,3]

Brain imaging studies of healthy subjects have estimated the incidence of incidental LGGs to be between 0.05% and 0.2% in the general population,[4–7] and a study of 4309 gliomas from the French Brain Tumor Study Bank revealed that 3% of LGG patients were asymptomatic at the time of diagnosis.[8] A study on the natural history of incidental gliomas demonstrated that if, not treated, these tumors become symptomatic at a median time of 48 months after diagnosis, typically with onset of seizures, or other neurologic signs such as hemiparesis; the same study showed these incidental gliomas grow at a rate of 3.5 mm per year as seen on radiological imaging.[9]

Disclosures: The authors have no commercial or financial conflicts of interest to declare.
[a] Department of Neurological Surgery, Barrow Neurological Institute, Saint Joseph's Hospital and Medical Center, 350 W Thomas Rd, Phoenix, AZ 85013, USA; [b] Department of Neurosurgery, Addenbrooke's Hospital, Hills Rd, Cambridge CB2 0QQ, UK
* Corresponding author.
E-mail address: Nader.Sanai@barrowbrainandspine.com

Moreover, incidental LGGs are proliferating at similar rates as symptomatic LGGs, with both tumor sets having a median Ki67 proliferative index of 5.0% in one study. Collectively, these findings suggest that incidental LGGs are an earlier phase in the natural history of LGGs.

GLIOMA GENETICS

The genetic basis of gliomas has been investigated intensively. The cell of origin of gliomas is currently unclear, but may be a neural stem cell or oligodendrocyte precursors.[10] Large-scale sequencing studies have been enormously helpful in elucidating a distinction in the genetic background of LGG compared with high-grade gliomas. Mutations in isocitrate dehydrogenase 1 (IDH1) are present in 80% of grade II and III gliomas and secondary glioblastomas, of which the IDH1 R132H mutation is most frequent.[11–16] In contrast, primary high-grade gliomas typically lack IDH1 mutations, and are more likely to have other genetic changes, such as mutations or amplifications in epidermal growth factor receptor.[17–19]

An important genetic alteration in LGG is that of p53, mutations in which are found in two-thirds of diffuse LGGs that later transform to more aggressive tumors.[20] The p53 gene is normally activated after DNA damage to cells, inducing transcription of genes whose ultimate effects include apoptosis. Mutations in p53 are thought to have effects such as inhibition of apoptosis, stimulation of cell proliferation, and neovascularization, which are hallmarks of cancer.[21]

It has been proposed that mutations in IDH1 are an early genetic event in LGGs that is followed by TERT promoter mutations and/or 1p/19q codeletions. Recent work has led to the classification of gliomas into 5 groups based on their status of TERT mutations, IDH mutations, and 1p/19q codeletion, with the best prognosis for TERT- and IDH-mutant tumors and triple-positive tumors, and the worst prognosis for gliomas that only have a TERT mutation.[22] To determine whether incidental LGGs harbor a similar mutational profile as LGGs and therefore are a part of a common natural history, a recent study analyzed for the presence of IDH1 mutations, TERT promoter mutations and 1p/19q codeletions in 23 incidental LGGs, and found these all occur with high frequency in this group of tumors.[23] This suggests that incidental LGGs and symptomatic LGGs share a common genetic basis.

DIAGNOSTIC IMAGING

The gold standard imaging modality for diagnosing LGGs is currently 1.5 T MRI (although 3-T MRI improves image resolution[24]), in which LGGs typically are isointense or hypointense on T1-weighted imaging and hyperintense on T2-weighted imaging, and usually do not enhance with contrast (although oligodendrogliomas do so in 25%–50% of cases). Because LGGs are slow growing, vasogenic edema and mass effect are less commonly seen on MRI. More recently, diffusion tensor imaging has emerged as a complementary imaging modality to structural MRI, because it can delineate functional tract deflection by tumors, which can certainly aid in preoperative planning to guide the optimal surgical approach and the resection margins. Intraoperative MRI scanning is being increasingly adopted for continuously assessing the progress of tumor resection during the operation and studies suggest that using MRI intraoperatively may enable increased extent of LGG resection with improved outcomes.[25–27]

Recent physiologic and metabolic imaging modalities can aid the diagnosis and targeting of LGGs.[28] In particular, proton MR spectroscopy is helpful in this regard by quantifying the distribution of cellular metabolite levels: a dominant choline peak (owing to higher membrane synthesis), low N-acetylaspartate (reflecting a reduced neuronal signature), and no lactate or lipid (owing to a lack of hypoxia or necrosis that is typical of high-grade gliomas), are characteristic of LGGs. This imaging modality can further guide biopsy target selection because the level of cellular proliferation in the tumor is correlated with the choline peak. The normalized creatinine/phosphocreatine levels of these tumors are also associated with both progression-free survival and malignant progression-free survival, thereby providing useful prognostic information.[29] At this point, however, it remains unproven whether MR spectroscopy is adequate for monitoring the progression of presumed LGGs.[30]

Another complementary imaging technique is PET scanning, which allows for quantification of tumor metabolism and therefore can help to guide biopsy location and identify histologic upgrading. LGGs are hypometabolic on PET imaging with 18F-fluorodeoxyglucose, in contrast with high-grade gliomas. Radiolabeled amino acids are increased in two-thirds of LGGs, and an example that is used by some in clinical practice is O-(2–18F-fluoroethyl)-L-tyrosine (FET).[31] In a retrospective study of 174 patients with new cerebral lesions, it was found that PET imaging with 18F-FET helped to differentiate gliomas from other lesions: a maximum tumor-to-brain ratio (TBR_{max}) of 18F-FET uptake above a threshold of 2.5 had 65% positive predictive value and 84% negative predictive value for detection of a tumor, supporting a further procedure such as biopsy or resection.[32] The TBR_{max} seems to increase with malignant progression of LGGs, and using TBR_{max} in addition to other parameters for PET imaging with 18F-FET (time–activity curve pattern of 18F uptake) was found to have a higher diagnostic accuracy for malignant progression than contrast enhancement on MRI, particularly with serial PET imaging with 18F-FET for dynamic information.[33–35]

STEREOTACTIC BIOPSY

Incidental gliomas are generally low grade, but histologic diagnosis is essential to confirm the diagnosis, for which tumor tissue can be obtained either via biopsy or from resection. The indications for biopsy of a suspected LGG are if the lesion is diffuse, such as gliomatosis, or the patient is medically unfit for a major operation of surgical tumor resection. A major disadvantage of histologic diagnosis from tissue obtained via biopsy is diagnostic inaccuracy owing to sampling error, which is particularly problematic in mixed gliomas and gliomas with low proliferative rates. Indeed, 28% of grade III gliomas are undergraded and 11% of grade II gliomas are overgraded from biopsy tissue alone.[36] As suggested, however, the diagnostic accuracy of biopsy can be improved significantly if complementary imaging approaches are used, such as PET imaging with 18F-fluorodeoxyglucose and proton MR spectroscopy, the latter of which can be performed at the time of routine brain MRI scanning and improves the diagnostic yield of biopsy for LGGs to close to 100%.[37–39] We anticipate these methodologies will become more widely used in this context as the technologies become more easily accessible.

MICROSURGICAL RESECTION

An important consideration for incidental gliomas is that these tumors tend to be significantly smaller at the time of diagnosis than LGGs. Moreover, they are also less likely to be situated near eloquent regions of the brain than their symptomatic counterparts.[9] These points offer a considerable advantage to the surgical management of incidental gliomas, in that they are more amenable to gross total resection. Comparing incidental and symptomatic LGG resections, a study reported gross total resection in 60% of incidental gliomas, much higher than the 31.5% rate for symptomatic LGGs.[40] Even in eloquent brain regions, it seems that incidental gliomas are more amenable to fuller resection: supratotal and total resections were achieved in 27% and 36%, respectively, in 1 report.[41] Accordingly, studies

have recently demonstrated improved overall survival in patients with resections for incidental glioma compared with those for LGGs.[9,23,40]

It is now well-established that the greater the extent of resection of LGGs, the better the long-term outcome for the patient. Several studies over the last few decades, using either volumetric or nonvolumetric tumor assessment, have evaluated the impact of extent of LGG resection on outcome, with the majority of studies demonstrating that the greater the extent of resection the better the overall survival and progression-free survival.[26,42–54] These results seem to apply both to hemispheric LGGs as well as to LGGs in limited to certain regions, for example, insular gliomas.[49,55] A review of the studies assessing the effect of extent of resection on outcomes has been published recently[56]; to summarize, 3 studies using volumetric assessment to determine the amount of resection for LGGs (462 patients in total) all showed increased 5-year survival with greater resection on univariate and/or multivariate analysis (**Table 1**),[26,51,52] with one of these studies also showing improved malignant progression-free survival.[51]

Recent analyses demonstrate survival benefits from more complete LGG resections are maintained in the very long term, even up to 10 years after the surgery.[51] When complete resections are achieved, the 10-year survival is close to 100%, but this progressively declines as the extent of resection decreases to 40% (**Fig. 1**).[51] It has also been demonstrated that leaving radiographically evident residual tumor tissue behind negatively impacts outcome, even if the original tumor is large. As imaging techniques become more advanced, the effects of resecting the last few percentile of LGG on patient outcome will become clearer, and this will be important in guiding neurosurgeons as to how aggressive they should be when resecting these tumors, particularly if they are adjacent to eloquent regions or tracts. To date, a volumetric "threshold" for LGG extent of resection remains unknown. A correlation between extent of resection of LGGs and survival may be related to biased treatment allocation, however. To exclude this, a retrospective analysis of 148 LGG patients showed eloquent location of the tumor was the strongest predictor of extent of resection, and the presence of a neurodeficit and extent of resection were the strongest predictors of overall survival, tumor recurrence, and malignant progression; importantly, after stratification by eloquent tumor location to correct for treatment bias, it was shown that extent of resection was still associated with improved overall survival.[57]

There is growing interest in the use of intraoperative MRI studies for improving the extent of

Table 1
Key studies using volumetric assessment of extent of resection for impact on survival in low grade gliomas patients

Study	No. of Patients	Extent of Resection, % (n)	5-y Survival (%)	5-y Overall Survival Univariate analysis P value	Multivariate analysis P value
Van Veelen et al,[52] 1998	90	>75 (13) <75 (59)	62 18	.002	.04
Claus et al,[26] 2005	156	100 (56) <100 (100)	98.2 92.0	.05	<.05
Smith et al,[51] 2008	216	0–40 (21) 41–69 (39) 70–89 (55) 90–98 (26) 100 (75)	NA NA NA 97.0 98.0	NA	<.001

Abbreviation: NA, not applicable.
Adapted from Hardesty DA, Sanai N. The value of glioma extent of resection in the modern neurosurgical era. Front Neurol 2012;3:140; with permission.

resection for LGGs. In a retrospective study of 102 patients undergoing LGG resection with the aid of intraoperative MRI, intraoperative MRI showed residual tumor present in 79 of these patients, of which 54 patients had tumor amenable for and underwent resection of this residual tumor volume.

Their data suggested therefore that intraoperative MRI improved the extent of resection, in particular for nonenhancing gliomas.[58] Similar results were confirmed in a multicenter, retrospective study of 288 patients for whom intraoperative MRI was used to guide LGG resection: gross total resection

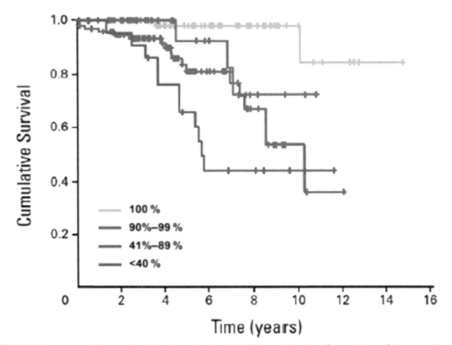

Fig. 1. Kaplan-Meier curves of overall patient survival with different levels of resection of low-grade glioma. The graph demonstrates stepwise improvement in survival with increasing extent of resection. (*Data from* Smith JS, Chang EF, Lamborn KR, et al. Role of extent of resection in the long-term outcome of low-grade hemispheric gliomas. J Clin Oncol 2008;26(8):1338–45; and *Adapted from* Sanai N, Chang S, and Berger MS. Low-grade gliomas in adults. J Neurosurg 2011;115(5):956, with permission.)

was found to be an independent prognostic factor for progression-free survival, and patients with residual tumor left inadvertently the prognosis was similar to those with partially resectable tumors.[59]

It is well-known that glioma cells infiltrate beyond the observed margins from T2-weighted MRI and/or fluid-attenuated inversion recovery imaging, in 1 study this infiltration was up to 26 mm beyond the observed margins on imaging.[60] Therefore, some have proposed a supratotal resection of LGGs in cases where the tumor is away from noneloquent regions, and this can alter the natural history by delaying malignant transformation in a subset of LGG.[60,61] Nevertheless, the optimal distance for resection beyond observable tumor margin remains debatable. In such cases where supratotal resection is preferred, intraoperative functional mapping is especially important for maximizing resection while minimizing risk of inducing neurologic deficits, particularly for incidental gliomas where operative morbidity must be kept to an absolute minimum. A recent analysis of long-term outcomes from supratotal resection for LGG, with 16 patients all with intraoperative mapping for supratotal resection (including a margin beyond fluid-attenuated inversion recovery-weighted MRI abnormalities) and a minimum of 8 years follow-up duration, showed that one-half of the patients had a recurrence but there were no cases of malignant progression or death even after such a long follow-up.[62] These data suggest the benefits of supratotal resection in cases without involvement of eloquent structures may be maintained in the long term, although more extensive and ideally prospective studies are required.

As discussed, molecular markers are known to have prognostic relevance for gliomas and these tumors can be stratified according to such markers as TERT mutations, IDH mutations, and 1p/19q codeletions.[22] This potentially creates a confounding factor for studies, suggesting that the extent of LGG resection improves outcome. To distinguish between these, a study looked at IDH1, p53, and 1p/19q status in 200 grade II gliomas that underwent resection, and demonstrated that a greater extent of resection was not attributable to tumors having favorable molecular markers and, therefore, that maximizing surgical resection independently predicts a better prognosis.[63]

FUNCTIONAL MAPPING

The benefits from more complete tumor resection of improved survival and delayed time to malignant progression must be balanced with the potential for neurologic deficits induced by damaging neighboring cortical tracts. Therefore, mapping of functional pathways during surgery for LGG is becoming increasingly common. For example, combining diffusion tensor tractography with the traditional MRI-based neuronavigation can reduce the likelihood of undesired damage to adjacent cortical tracts and thus neurologic deficits. Indeed, in an analysis of 238 glioma patients randomized to diffusion tensor tractography or MRI neuronavigation without diffusion tensor tractography, the former had a lower rate of postoperative motor deficits (15.3%) compared with the latter (32.8%).[64]

For LGGs adjacent to eloquent motor areas such as the rolandic cortex, there is clearly a greater risk of damaging descending motor pathways and inducing motor deficits. In these instances, intraoperative cortical stimulation mapping can be hugely influential in guiding the surgeon toward the limits of resection by defining the boundaries of the motor tracts.[65–67] A study that used cortical stimulation mapping and achieved gross total resection in 46.1% of LGG cases found that immediate postoperative deficits were in 59.3% of patients in whom a subcortical motor tract was demonstrated intraoperatively, but only in 10.9% of patients where this was not demonstrated (although permanent deficits were in 6.5% and 3.5%, respectively).[65] Another publication reporting the use of cortical stimulation mapping in which 87% gross total or subtotal LGG resection was achieved, yielded neurologic morbidity in only 5% of cases.[66] Hence, the data suggest that stimulation mapping is helpful in LGG resection when there is a risk of damaging motor pathways.

Intraoperative stimulation mapping is also very helpful if there is a possibility that the tumor may be situated within or adjacent to eloquent language cortex. This is especially true because, in contrast with motor areas, which are more consistent in their location, language regions tend to vary significantly from 1 patient to the next, making predictions on their specific locations difficult without stimulation mapping.[68] For example, the distance between the temporal pole and the temporal language area varies from 3 to 9 cm,[69] and similarly for the inferior frontal region the language area often extends beyond the traditional Broca's area.[68] Another level of complexity is added by the finding that functional language cortex may be located within the tumor itself, such that it may not necessarily be safe to debulk the tumor from within.[70] A report of 243 surviving patients after glioma resection in which intraoperative language mapping was used found that 4 patients (1.6%) had a lasting new language deficit 6 months after surgery, and that the gross total resection rate was 51.6% in the LGG cohort.[68] This finding suggests that intraoperative language mapping effectively minimizes inducing language deficits while maximizing the extent of resection for LGGs. Interestingly, the recent UCSF Low-Grade Glioma Scoring system incorporates area of eloquence as 1 of 4 prognostic factors,[71] and this system has been validated externally,[72] further supporting the importance of intraoperative cortical stimulation mapping for these tumors. Some have even argued for combined diffusion tensor imaging-based identification of tracts with intraoperative motor and language mapping for tumor resection.[73]

Given that neurocognitive defects tend to be more difficult to diagnose than pure motor deficits, there is increasing realization of the importance of establishing a baseline of cognition preoperatively. A study using comprehensive neuropsychological testing preoperatively and postoperatively for 22 LGG patients undergoing resection with awake mapping found that 55% of patients had new transient or mild neurocognitive deficits. The language deficits tended to be stable or improved, whereas some patients showed a decline in performance in memory tasks. Therefore, awake mapping seems to provide promising outcomes for language for tumors in eloquent cortex, although cognitive assessments at baseline are needed to determine the real impact of resection on cognition, especially on memory.[74] A useful example of where cortical and subcortical intraoperative mapping can help to preserve cognitive function during LGG resection is from a recent study of 8 patients with tumors in the left sagittal stratum, a region with complex functional anatomy comprising several important tracts for language and vision. Subcortical stimulation of the sagittal stratum induced transient deficits such as semantic paraphasia, alexia, and phonemic paraphasia owing to the presence of various functional tracts. In all patients, the resection was terminated at limits defined by these functional borders, and postoperatively there were no permanent language deficits, highlighting the usefulness of intraoperative mapping particularly in functionally complex eloquent areas.[75] Even though incidental LGG patients do not report symptoms attributable to the tumor, a study reported 60% of these patients have neuropsychological disturbances as demonstrated on detailed assessment: 53% with executive dysfunction, 20% with working memory impairment, and 6% with attentional disturbances. This further argues in favor of careful preoperative neuropsychological assessment to establish a baseline, with surgical mapping being used as necessary for tumors in eloquent locations to avoid inducing cognitive deficits in incidental LGGs.[76]

MALIGNANT TRANSFORMATION

The prognosis dramatically worsens when an LGG undergoes malignant transformation or histologic upgrading, which is reported to occur at a median interval of between 2.1 and 10.1 years.[44,51,77–80] The risk of LGG transformation is significant, although incidences are highly variable in reports, varying from 17% to 73%.[44,51,77,79,81–85] There is evidence suggesting that larger tumors are more likely to undergo transformation sooner than smaller tumors, possibly because larger size reflects a higher baseline proliferative rate of tumor cells; these tumors may have faster recurrence after complete resections.[51] This growth rate of LGGs seems to impact survival: a study of 143 LGG patients reported that a tumor growth rate of 8 mm or more per year was associated with a shorter median survival of 5.1 years in comparison with a 15.0-year survival when the growth rate was less than 8 mm per year.[86] Using serial imaging to detect tumors with faster growth rates can thus be useful for identifying patients with a greater risk of malignant transformation.[87] Importantly, it is increasingly appreciated that the extent of surgical resection has a significant impact on the risk of transformation, with greater resections lowering this risk for both hemispheric LGG and insular LGGs: the volume of residual tumor is a predictor of transformation.[49] A study of 191 LGG patients undergoing resection reported a 5-year malignancy-free survival rate of 74%, with 3 independent associated with malignant transformation: fibrillary astrocytoma pathology (relative risk, 1.8), tumor size (relative risk, 1.086), and gross total resection (relative risk, 0.526).[77] These data argue against a conservative management approach of 'watching and waiting' after a simple biopsy, and strongly favor a move toward more aggressive early intervention to maximize the extent of surgical resection if the patient is medically fit for this operation. Indeed, an interesting case was reported of a patient with an incidental LGG who was treated conservatively, with yearly MRI scans showing slow growth over 6 years until there was a rapid acceleration of growth suggesting malignant transformation, prompting surgical resection that demonstrated glioblastoma.[88] This patient was still asymptomatic at the time of resection, suggesting an absence of symptoms does not exclude transformation for incidental LGGs, and supporting the role of earlier resections in incidental LGGs as well.

It must be noted, however, that greater extent of resection may not delay malignant progression for all LGGs. A study of 93 patients with grade II oligodendrogliomas found that having a larger resection improved overall survival and progression-free survival but did not delay malignant progression for this particular tumor subtype (despite controlling for 1p/19q codeletion).[89]

ADVANCED TECHNOLOGIES

In high-grade gliomas, it has been demonstrated that protoporphyrin IX accumulates in tumor tissue more so than normal brain, and this can be visualized by fluorescence when 5-aminolevulinic acid (5-ALA) is administered to the patient. This allows for fluorescence-guided resections of glioblastoma, which can improve the extent of resection by helping to distinguish the brain–tumor interface. In contrast with high-grade gliomas, however, the use of 5-ALA–guided resections for LGGs is less well-established. By comparing the fluorescence induced by 5-ALA in 12 LGG patients undergoing resection with the histopathology, a recent study demonstrated that visible fluorescence had a poor diagnostic accuracy of only 38.0%, but that this could be improved to 67.0% if quantitative fluorescence was used (and this approaches the diagnostic accuracy of visible fluorescence in high-grade gliomas).[90] Another way of potentially increasing the diagnostic accuracy of 5-ALA for fluorescence guided resections of LGGs is to use intraoperative confocal microscopy, which may allow visualization of fluorescence at the tumor cellular level, although more data are awaited regarding its benefit in clinical practice.[91,92] It has also been found that 5-ALA fluorescence correlates with tumor proliferative (Ki-67) index and high-grade pathology,[93] suggesting that areas of fluorescence seen in LGG may be those at risk of transformation and, therefore, requiring a more aggressive resection if feasible.

SUMMARY

Incidentally discovered gliomas are likely to be an early part of the natural history of gliomas, and most are LGG. Although further studies are required to add data for more patients on outcomes after resections of incidental gliomas, current evidence points toward a rationale for an early maximal resection where possible to improve survival and potentially delay onset of malignant progression, as is the case for symptomatic LGG. The use of novel technologies, including diffusion tensor imaging, FET-PET or PET with 18F-fluorodeoxyglucose imaging, and intraoperative mapping of motor and language tracts may greatly aid in ensuring maximal resections while minimizing any cognitive, motor, or sensory postoperative deficits, which is particularly important in this group of patients who are asymptomatic at the time of diagnosis.

REFERENCES

1. Kurzwelly D, Herrlinger U, Simon M. Seizures in patients with low-grade gliomas–incidence, pathogenesis, surgical management, and pharmacotherapy. Adv Tech Stand Neurosurg 2010;35:81–111.
2. Mandonnet E, de Witt Hamer P, Pallud J, et al. Silent diffuse low-grade glioma: toward screening and preventive treatment? Cancer 2014;120(12):1758–62.
3. Pallud J, Capelle L, Taillandier L, et al. The silent phase of diffuse low-grade gliomas. Is it when we missed the action? Acta Neurochir (Wien) 2013;155(12):2237–42.
4. Katzman GL, Dagher AP, Patronas NJ. Incidental findings on brain magnetic resonance imaging from 1000 asymptomatic volunteers. JAMA 1999;282(1):36–9.
5. Onizuka M, Suyama K, Shibayama A, et al. Asymptomatic brain tumor detected at brain check-up. Neurol Med Chir (Tokyo) 2001;41(9):431–4 [discussion: 435].
6. Vernooij MW, Ikram MA, Tanghe HL, et al. Incidental findings on brain MRI in the general population. N Engl J Med 2007;357(18):1821–8.
7. Weber F, Knopf H. Incidental findings in magnetic resonance imaging of the brains of healthy young men. J Neurol Sci 2006;240(1–2):81–4.
8. Bauchet L, Rigau V, Mathieu-Daudé H, et al. French brain tumor data bank: methodology and first results on 10,000 cases. J Neurooncol 2007;84(2):189–99.
9. Pallud J, Fontaine D, Duffau H, et al. Natural history of incidental World Health Organization grade II gliomas. Ann Neurol 2010;68(5):727–33.
10. Liu C, Sage JC, Miller MR, et al. Mosaic analysis with double markers reveals tumor cell of origin in glioma. Cell 2011;146(2):209–21.
11. Balss J, Meyer J, Mueller W, et al. Analysis of the IDH1 codon 132 mutation in brain tumors. Acta Neuropathol 2008;116(6):597–602.
12. Hartmann C, Meyer J, Balss J, et al. Type and frequency of IDH1 and IDH2 mutations are related to astrocytic and oligodendroglial differentiation and age: a study of 1,010 diffuse gliomas. Acta Neuropathol 2009;118(4):469–74.
13. Yan H, Parsons DW, Jin G, et al. IDH1 and IDH2 mutations in gliomas. N Engl J Med 2009;360(8):765–73.
14. Sanson M, Marie Y, Paris S, et al. Isocitrate dehydrogenase 1 codon 132 mutation is an important prognostic biomarker in gliomas. J Clin Oncol 2009;27(25):4150–4.
15. Watanabe T, Nobusawa S, Kleihues P, et al. IDH1 mutations are early events in the development of astrocytomas and oligodendrogliomas. Am J Pathol 2009;174(4):1149–53.

16. Bleeker FE, Lamba S, Leenstra S, et al. IDH1 mutations at residue p.R132 (IDH1(R132)) occur frequently in high-grade gliomas but not in other solid tumors. Hum Mutat 2009;30(1):7–11.

17. Cancer Genome Atlas Research Network. Comprehensive genomic characterization defines human glioblastoma genes and core pathways. Nature 2008;455(7216):1061–8.

18. Verhaak RG, Hoadley KA, Purdom E, et al. Integrated genomic analysis identifies clinically relevant subtypes of glioblastoma characterized by abnormalities in PDGFRA, IDH1, EGFR, and NF1. Cancer Cell 2010;17(1):98–110.

19. Parsons DW, Jones S, Zhang X, et al. An integrated genomic analysis of human glioblastoma multiforme. Science 2008;321(5897):1807–12.

20. Ohgaki H, Dessen P, Jourde B, et al. Genetic pathways to glioblastoma: a population-based study. Cancer Res 2004;64(19):6892–9.

21. Hanahan D, Weinberg RA. Hallmarks of cancer: the next generation. Cell 2011;144(5):646–74.

22. Eckel-Passow JE, Lachance DH, Molinaro AM, et al. Glioma Groups Based on 1p/19q, IDH, and TERT Promoter Mutations in Tumors. N Engl J Med 2015; 372(26):2499–508.

23. Zhang ZY, Chan AK, Ng HK, et al. Surgically treated incidentally discovered low-grade gliomas are mostly IDH mutated and 1p19q co-deleted with favorable prognosis. Int J Clin Exp Pathol 2014; 7(12):8627–36.

24. Pamir MN, Ozduman K, Dinçer A, et al. First intraoperative, shared-resource, ultrahigh-field 3-Tesla magnetic resonance imaging system and its application in low-grade glioma resection. J Neurosurg 2010;112(1):57–69.

25. Black PM, Alexander E 3rd, Martin C, et al. Craniotomy for tumor treatment in an intraoperative magnetic resonance imaging unit. Neurosurgery 1999; 45(3):423–31 [discussion: 431–3].

26. Claus EB, Horlacher A, Hsu L, et al. Survival rates in patients with low-grade glioma after intraoperative magnetic resonance image guidance. Cancer 2005;103(6):1227–33.

27. Pamir MN, Ozduman K. 3-T ultrahigh-field intraoperative MRI for low-grade glioma resection. Expert Rev Anticancer Ther 2009;9(11):1537–9.

28. Chang SM, Nelson S, Vandenberg S, et al. Integration of preoperative anatomic and metabolic physiologic imaging of newly diagnosed glioma. J Neurooncol 2009;92(3):401–15.

29. Hattingen E, Raab P, Franz K, et al. Prognostic value of choline and creatine in WHO grade II gliomas. Neuroradiology 2008;50(9):759–67.

30. Reijneveld JC, van der Grond J, Ramos LM, et al. Proton MRS imaging in the follow-up of patients with suspected low-grade gliomas. Neuroradiology 2005;47(12):887–91.

31. Floeth FW, Pauleit D, Sabel M, et al. Prognostic value of O-(2-18F-fluoroethyl)-L-tyrosine PET and MRI in low-grade glioma. J Nucl Med 2007;48(4):519–27.

32. Rapp M, Heinzel A, Galldiks N, et al. Diagnostic performance of 18F-FET PET in newly diagnosed cerebral lesions suggestive of glioma. J Nucl Med 2013;54(2):229–35.

33. Galldiks N, Stoffels G, Ruge MI, et al. Role of O-(2-18F-fluoroethyl)-L-tyrosine PET as a diagnostic tool for detection of malignant progression in patients with low-grade glioma. J Nucl Med 2013;54(12): 2046–54.

34. Galldiks N, Stoffels G, Filss C, et al. The use of dynamic O-(2-18F-fluoroethyl)-l-tyrosine PET in the diagnosis of patients with progressive and recurrent glioma. Neuro Oncol 2015;17(9):1293–300.

35. Jansen NL, Suchorska B, Wenter V, et al. Dynamic 18F-FET PET in newly diagnosed astrocytic low-grade glioma identifies high-risk patients. J Nucl Med 2014;55(2):198–203.

36. Muragaki Y, Chernov M, Maruyama T, et al. Low-grade glioma on stereotactic biopsy: how often is the diagnosis accurate? Minim Invasive Neurosurg 2008;51(5):275–9.

37. Hall WA, Martin A, Liu H, et al. Improving diagnostic yield in brain biopsy: coupling spectroscopic targeting with real-time needle placement. J Magn Reson Imaging 2001;13(1):12–5.

38. Martin AJ, Liu H, Hall WA, et al. Preliminary assessment of turbo spectroscopic imaging for targeting in brain biopsy. AJNR Am J Neuroradiol 2001;22(5): 959–68.

39. Chernov MF, Muragaki Y, Ochiai T, et al. Spectroscopy-supported frame-based image-guided stereotactic biopsy of parenchymal brain lesions: comparative evaluation of diagnostic yield and diagnostic accuracy. Clin Neurol Neurosurg 2009; 111(6):527–35.

40. Potts MB, Smith JS, Molinaro AM, et al. Natural history and surgical management of incidentally discovered low-grade gliomas. J Neurosurg 2012; 116(2):365–72.

41. Duffau H. Awake surgery for incidental WHO grade II gliomas involving eloquent areas. Acta Neurochir (Wien) 2012;154(4):575–84 [discussion: 584].

42. Johannesen TB, Langmark F, Lote K. Progress in long-term survival in adult patients with supratentorial low-grade gliomas: a population-based study of 993 patients in whom tumors were diagnosed between 1970 and 1993. J Neurosurg 2003;99(5): 854–62.

43. Leighton C, Fisher B, Bauman G, et al. Supratentorial low-grade glioma in adults: an analysis of prognostic factors and timing of radiation. J Clin Oncol 1997;15(4):1294–301.

44. McGirt MJ, Chaichana KL, Attenello FJ, et al. Extent of surgical resection is independently associated

with survival in patients with hemispheric infiltrating low-grade gliomas. Neurosurgery 2008;63(4):700–7 [author reply: 707–8].

45. Nakamura M, Konishi N, Tsunoda S, et al. Analysis of prognostic and survival factors related to treatment of low-grade astrocytomas in adults. Oncology 2000;58(2):108–16.

46. North CA, North RB, Epstein JA, et al. Low-grade cerebral astrocytomas. Survival and quality of life after radiation therapy. Cancer 1990;66(1):6–14.

47. Philippon JH, Clemenceau SH, Fauchon FH, et al. Supratentorial low-grade astrocytomas in adults. Neurosurgery 1993;32(4):554–9.

48. Ahmadi R, Dictus C, Hartmann C, et al. Long-term outcome and survival of surgically treated supratentorial low-grade glioma in adult patients. Acta Neurochir (Wien) 2009;151(11):1359–65.

49. Sanai N, Polley MY, Berger MS. Insular glioma resection: assessment of patient morbidity, survival, and tumor progression. J Neurosurg 2010;112(1):1–9.

50. Shaw EG, Berkey B, Coons SW, et al. Recurrence following neurosurgeon-determined gross-total resection of adult supratentorial low-grade glioma: results of a prospective clinical trial. J Neurosurg 2008;109(5):835–41.

51. Smith JS, Chang EF, Lamborn KR, et al. Role of extent of resection in the long-term outcome of low-grade hemispheric gliomas. J Clin Oncol 2008; 26(8):1338–45.

52. van Veelen ML, Avezaat CJ, Kros JM, et al. Supratentorial low grade astrocytoma: prognostic factors, dedifferentiation, and the issue of early versus late surgery. J Neurol Neurosurg Psychiatry 1998;64(5):581–7.

53. Whitton AC, Bloom HJ. Low grade glioma of the cerebral hemispheres in adults: a retrospective analysis of 88 cases. Int J Radiat Oncol Biol Phys 1990;18(4):783–6.

54. Sanai N, Berger MS. Glioma extent of resection and its impact on patient outcome. Neurosurgery 2008; 62(4):753–64 [discussion: 264–6].

55. Simon M, Neuloh G, von Lehe M, et al. Insular gliomas: the case for surgical management. J Neurosurg 2009;110(4):685–95.

56. Hardesty DA, Sanai N. The value of glioma extent of resection in the modern neurosurgical era. Front Neurol 2012;3:140.

57. Gousias K, Schramm J, Simon M. Extent of resection and survival in supratentorial infiltrative low-grade gliomas: analysis of and adjustment for treatment bias. Acta Neurochir (Wien) 2014;156(2):327–37.

58. Mohammadi AM, Sullivan TB, Barnett GH, et al. Use of high-field intraoperative magnetic resonance imaging to enhance the extent of resection of enhancing and nonenhancing gliomas. Neurosurgery 2014;74(4): 339–48 [discussion: 349; quiz 349–50].

59. Coburger J, Merkel A, Scherer M, et al. Low-grade glioma surgery in intraoperative magnetic resonance imaging: results of a multicenter retrospective assessment of the German Study Group for intraoperative Magnetic Resonance Imaging. Neurosurgery 2016;78(6):775–86.

60. Pallud J, Varlet P, Devaux B, et al. Diffuse low-grade oligodendrogliomas extend beyond MRI-defined abnormalities. Neurology 2010;74(21):1724–31.

61. Yordanova YN, Moritz-Gasser S, Duffau H. Awake surgery for WHO Grade II gliomas within "noneloquent" areas in the left dominant hemisphere: toward a "supratotal" resection. Clinical article. J Neurosurg 2011;115(2):232–9.

62. Duffau H. Long-term outcomes after supratotal resection of diffuse low-grade gliomas: a consecutive series with 11-year follow-up. Acta Neurochir (Wien) 2016;158(1):51–8.

63. Cordier D, Gozé C, Schädelin S, et al. A better surgical resectability of WHO grade II gliomas is independent of favorable molecular markers. J Neurooncol 2015;121(1):185–93.

64. Wu JS, Zhou LF, Tang WJ, et al. Clinical evaluation and follow-up outcome of diffusion tensor imaging-based functional neuronavigation: a prospective, controlled study in patients with gliomas involving pyramidal tracts. Neurosurgery 2007;61(5):935–48 [discussion: 948–9].

65. Carrabba G, Fava E, Giussani C, et al. Cortical and subcortical motor mapping in rolandic and perirolandic glioma surgery: impact on postoperative morbidity and extent of resection. J Neurosurg Sci 2007;51(2):45–51.

66. Duffau H, Capelle L, Sichez J, et al. Intra-operative direct electrical stimulations of the central nervous system: the Salpetriere experience with 60 patients. Acta Neurochir (Wien) 1999;141(11):1157–67.

67. Keles GE, Lundin DA, Lamborn KR, et al. Intraoperative subcortical stimulation mapping for hemispherical perirolandic gliomas located within or adjacent to the descending motor pathways: evaluation of morbidity and assessment of functional outcome in 294 patients. J Neurosurg 2004; 100(3):369–75.

68. Sanai N, Mirzadeh Z, Berger MS. Functional outcome after language mapping for glioma resection. N Engl J Med 2008;358(1):18–27.

69. Ojemann G, Ojemann J, Lettich E, et al. Cortical language localization in left, dominant hemisphere. An electrical stimulation mapping investigation in 117 patients. J Neurosurg 1989;71(3):316–26.

70. Skirboll SS, Ojemann GA, Berger MS, et al. Functional cortex and subcortical white matter located within gliomas. Neurosurgery 1996;38(4):678–84 [discussion: 684–5].

71. Chang EF, Smith JS, Chang SM, et al. Preoperative prognostic classification system for hemispheric low-grade gliomas in adults. J Neurosurg 2008; 109(5):817–24.

72. Chang EF, Clark A, Jensen RL, et al. Multiinstitutional validation of the University of California at San Francisco Low-Grade Glioma Prognostic Scoring System. Clinical article. J Neurosurg 2009;111(2):203–10.

73. Bello L, Gambini A, Castellano A, et al. Motor and language DTI Fiber Tracking combined with intraoperative subcortical mapping for surgical removal of gliomas. Neuroimage 2008;39(1):369–82.

74. Racine CA, Li J, Molinaro AM, et al. Neurocognitive function in newly diagnosed low-grade glioma patients undergoing surgical resection with awake mapping techniques. Neurosurgery 2015;77(3):371–9 [discussion: 379].

75. Chan-Seng E, Moritz-Gasser S, Duffau H. Awake mapping for low-grade gliomas involving the left sagittal stratum: anatomofunctional and surgical considerations. J Neurosurg 2014;120(5):1069–77.

76. Cochereau J, Herbet G, Duffau H. Patients with incidental WHO grade II glioma frequently suffer from neuropsychological disturbances. Acta Neurochir (Wien) 2016;158(2):305–12.

77. Chaichana KL, McGirt MJ, Laterra J, et al. Recurrence and malignant degeneration after resection of adult hemispheric low-grade gliomas. J Neurosurg 2010;112(1):10–7.

78. Kreth FW, Warnke PC, Ostertag CB. Low grade supratentorial astrocytomas: management and prognostic factors. Cancer 1994;74(12):3247–8.

79. Lote K, Egeland T, Hager B, et al. Survival, prognostic factors, and therapeutic efficacy in low-grade glioma: a retrospective study in 379 patients. J Clin Oncol 1997;15(9):3129–40.

80. Shafqat S, Hedley-Whyte ET, Henson JW. Age-dependent rate of anaplastic transformation in low-grade astrocytoma. Neurology 1999;52(4):867–9.

81. Afra D, Osztie E. Histologically confirmed changes on CT of reoperated low-grade astrocytomas. Neuroradiology 1997;39(11):804–10.

82. Janny P, Cure H, Mohr M, et al. Low grade supratentorial astrocytomas. Management and prognostic factors. Cancer 1994;73(7):1937–45.

83. Dirks PB, Jay V, Becker LE, et al. Development of anaplastic changes in low-grade astrocytomas of childhood. Neurosurgery 1994;34(1):68–78.

84. Lunsford LD, Somaza S, Kondziolka D, et al. Survival after stereotactic biopsy and irradiation of cerebral nonanaplastic, nonpilocytic astrocytoma. J Neurosurg 1995;82(4):523–9.

85. Piepmeier J, Christopher S, Spencer D, et al. Variations in the natural history and survival of patients with supratentorial low-grade astrocytomas. Neurosurgery 1996;38(5):872–8 [discussion: 878–9].

86. Pallud J, Mandonnet E, Duffau H, et al. Prognostic value of initial magnetic resonance imaging growth rates for World Health Organization grade II gliomas. Ann Neurol 2006;60(3):380–3.

87. Rees J, Watt H, Jäger HR, et al. Volumes and growth rates of untreated adult low-grade gliomas indicate risk of early malignant transformation. Eur J Radiol 2009;72(1):54–64.

88. Cochereau J, Herbet G, Rigau V, et al. Acute progression of untreated incidental WHO Grade II glioma to glioblastoma in an asymptomatic patient. J Neurosurg 2016;124(1):141–5.

89. Snyder LA, Wolf AB, Oppenlander ME, et al. The impact of extent of resection on malignant transformation of pure oligodendrogliomas. J Neurosurg 2014;120(2):309–14.

90. Valdes PA, Jacobs V, Harris BT, et al. Quantitative fluorescence using 5-aminolevulinic acid-induced protoporphyrin IX biomarker as a surgical adjunct in low-grade glioma surgery. J Neurosurg 2015;123(3):771–80.

91. Sanai N, Snyder LA, Honea NJ, et al. Intraoperative confocal microscopy in the visualization of 5-aminolevulinic acid fluorescence in low-grade gliomas. J Neurosurg 2011;115(4):740–8.

92. Meza D, Wang D, Wang Y, et al. Comparing high-resolution microscopy techniques for potential intraoperative use in guiding low-grade glioma resections. Lasers Surg Med 2015;47(4):289–95.

93. Jaber M, Wölfer J, Ewelt C, et al. The value of 5-Aminolevulinic acid in low-grade gliomas and high-grade gliomas lacking glioblastoma imaging features: an analysis based on fluorescence, Magnetic Resonance Imaging, 18F-Fluoroethyl tyrosine positron emission tomography, and tumor molecular factors. Neurosurgery 2016;78(3):401–11 [discussion: 411].

Reoperation for Recurrent Glioblastoma Multiforme

Adam M. Robin, MS, MD[a], Ian Lee, MD[b],
Steven N. Kalkanis, MD[b],*

KEYWORDS

- Glioblastoma multiforme • Resection • Recurrence • Reoperation • Extent of resection • Survival

KEY POINTS

- It is not known whether repeated operations for recurrent glioblastoma multiforme impart any benefit to patients with this disease.
- There are no high-quality data to guide neurosurgeons in the treatment of recurrent glioblastoma.
- Available data suggest that there may be some survival advantage depending on the degree of resection, both initial and repeat.
- Additionally, repeat operations may enhance survival and provide opportunities for patients to enroll in clinical trials, thus, potentially improving care contemporaneously and for future patients.

INTRODUCTION

The hallmark of glioblastoma multiforme (GBM) is its penchant for relentless progression. The median progression-free survival (PFS) is 4.4 to 8.4 months in patients with newly diagnosed GBM following the current standard of care, safely obtained maximal resection at initial surgery followed by concomitant temozolomide (TMZ) and radiotherapy and adjuvant TMZ.[1–3] In the highly favorable patient population typically garnered for clinical trials research, some patients have seen significantly improved median overall survival (mOS) to 20.5 months.[3] However, not all patients are eligible for clinical trial involvement, let alone surgery with a goal of complete resection. Indeed, it has been estimated that less than half of patients presenting with GBM receive an operation for resection owing to inoperability of the tumor or the poor surgical candidacy of the patient.[4,5]

The situation is even more dire for patients with recurrent GBM as rates of reoperation range from 3% to 30%.[6–10] Some evidence supports reoperation in select individuals with accessible focal tumors, younger age, and higher performance status (PS) in which a complete or near complete resection of the enhancing tumor can be achieved.[10–18] Nevertheless, there is also significant data indicating no benefit of reoperation, particularly when controlling for these prognostic variables and others.[19–23] Despite evidence-based guidelines and review articles focused on the role of reoperation for recurrent or progressive disease, repeat surgery remains controversial.[10,15,16,24–26] Several well-written reviews have been published in the last several years, but none focused on patients predominantly treated in the modern neuro-oncology era or inclusive of the relative surge in studies published over the last 3 to 4 years on this topic. Further evaluation and literature review is, therefore, warranted; herein the

Disclosure Statement: The authors have nothing to disclose.
[a] Department of Neurosurgery, Memorial Sloan Kettering Cancer Center, 1275 York Avenue, New York, NY 10065, USA; [b] Department of Neurosurgery, Henry Ford Hospital, 2799 West Grand Boulevard, Detroit, MI 48202, USA
* Corresponding author. Department of Neurosurgery, Henry Ford Hospital, K-11, 2799 West Grand Boulevard, Detroit, MI 48202.
E-mail address: Skalkan1@hfhs.org

Neurosurg Clin N Am 28 (2017) 407–428
http://dx.doi.org/10.1016/j.nec.2017.02.007
1042-3680/17/© 2017 Elsevier Inc. All rights reserved.

authors seek to identify the current available contemporary evidence, report on its conclusions, and reconcile the data when possible.

METHODS

The authors sought to determine the role of reoperation in extending survival for patients with progressive or recurrent GBM in the modern neuro-oncology era. The modern neuro-oncology era was defined as the era since wide recognition and adoption of radiotherapy plus concomitant and adjuvant TMZ and includes studies published since 2005 and excludes studies whereby recruitment of patients precedes 1995.[27,28] A comprehensive literature review was undertaken using Medline, Embase, Cochrane Library, and Web of Science. These databases were queried for English-language articles published since 2005 based on the following search strategies (accessed August 26, 2016):

PubMed
("glioblastoma multiforme" OR GBM OR "Glioblastoma"[Mesh]) AND (recurrence OR "Recurrence"[Mesh] OR "Neoplasm Recurrence, Local"[Mesh]) AND (reoperation OR resection OR "repeat operation" OR "Reoperation"[Mesh] OR "Second-Look Surgery"[Mesh])

Embase
'glioblastoma multiforme'/exp OR 'glioblastoma multiforme' OR gbm OR glioblastoma OR 'glioblastoma'/exp AND ('recurrence'/exp OR recurrence OR 'cancer recurrence'/exp OR 'recurrent disease'/exp) AND ('reoperation'/exp OR reoperation OR 'repeat resection' OR (resection AND repeat) OR 'repeat operation') AND [adult]/lim AND [English]/lim AND [2005–2016]/py

Cochrane
('glioblastoma multiforme' or GBM or glioblastoma) and (recurrence) and (reoperation or 'repeat resection' or 're-resection' or (resection and repeat) or 'repeat operation')

Web of Science
("glioblastoma multiforme" OR GBM) AND (recurrence) AND (reoperation OR "repeat resection" OR "re-resection" OR (resection AND repeat) OR "repeat operation") NOT (elderly OR geriatric OR 65 + OR "over 65")

After first-stage record screen, bibliographic review of the remaining full-text articles was conducted. Studies were evaluated for design, inclusion and exclusion criteria, number of patients, mOS, mOS following reoperation for recurrent GBM (rOS), PFS from initial surgery (PFS1), PFS following reoperation for recurrent GBM (PFS2), quality of life and/or performance status, indications for reoperation, inclusion and exclusion criteria, and for prognostic factors deemed important to survival.

RESULTS

Two hundred twenty-five records were identified via PubMed, Embase, Cochrane Library, and Web of Science database review (**Fig. 1**). The first author conducted a first-stage screening of the initial 225 records. One hundred sixty-nine records were excluded for the following reasons: duplicative results (n = 56), full-text article in language other than English (n = 11), other neoplasm (n = 27), chemotherapy or radiotherapy only (n = 15), case report or case series consisting of surgical series less than 20 patients (n = 20), or review article only (n = 40). A total of 56 full-text records then underwent second-stage review. Further exclusions were made for being mixed histology analyses (World Health Organization III and IV) (n = 6), surgery for newly diagnosed GBM (n = 3), clinical trials primarily evaluating brachytherapy, convection-enhanced delivery, or immunotherapy (n = 18). Only primary studies including reoperation for recurrent GBM published in full English text were retained for further evaluation. Reference review of this group yielded an additional 4 studies for final inclusion. A total of 33 articles were evaluated (**Table 1**).

Most studies were retrospective in nature (n = 27). However, 6 studies were either conducted prospectively or were derived from prospectively collected databases/post hoc analysis of clinical trial data (**Table 2**). There were no randomized controlled trials. Most of the data supported a role for reoperation in the treatment of recurrent or progressive GBM (n = 20). Ten studies either saw no evidence for a benefit of reoperation or suggested alternative treatment strategies (eg, multimodality treatment or stereotactic radiosurgery with or without TMZ). Sixteen articles considered the extent of resection (EOR) as a factor in survival. In total, 2717 patients who underwent a reoperation for progressive or recurrent GBM are accounted for in the authors' analysis. Two hundred fifty-eight patients had a second reoperation and 78 patients had 3 or more reoperations. Twelve studies reported on adjuvant therapies following resection. About half of the investigators reported on perioperative complications (**Table 3**) and their indications for reoperation (**Table 4**). Inclusion criteria for involvement in each study were explicitly given in all studies reviewed. The reported mOS from each study was averaged for all patients from initial diagnosis and from reoperation/recurrence and noted to be 19.1 (21 studies) and 9.9 (19 studies)

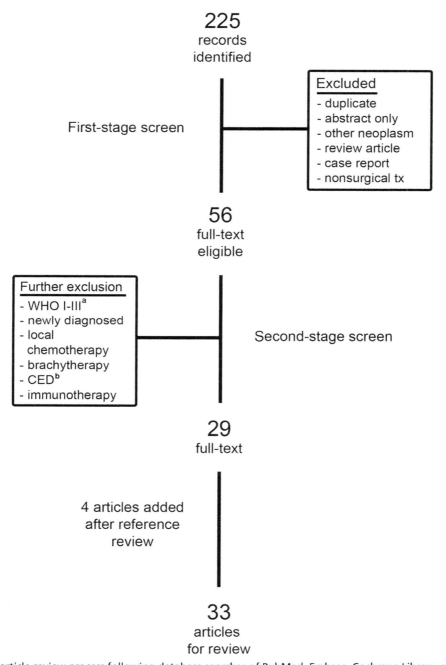

Fig. 1. The article review process following database searches of PubMed, Embase, Cochrane Library, and Web of Science. [a]World Health Organization (WHO) I to III, WHO glioma grades I to III, [b]CED, convection-enhanced delivery.

months, respectively (**Table 5**). The approximate mean complication rate is 18.9%.

DISCUSSION
Inclusion and Exclusion Criteria

All investigators required neuropathology diagnosis of GBM at initial surgery and on recurrence.

In cases of post hoc analysis of clinical trial data, central neuroradiology review was also required. In general, other inclusion criteria include an age greater than 18 years, complete records available for review, Karnofsky performance scale (KPS) 50 to 80 or greater, Eastern Cooperative Oncology Group (ECOG) scale 0 to 2, supratentorial location, focal lesion, de novo GBM status, and

Table 1
Study description and conclusions

Study/year	Study Description	Study Conclusions
Archavalis et al,[62] 2014	Comparison of varying combination salvage therapies in recurrent GBM: group 1: reoperation and HDR brachytherapy + TMZ (n = 20); group 2: HDR-brachytherapy + TMZ (n = 26); group 3: resurgery + TMZ (n = 20) vs an historical control of dose dense TMZ (n = 24)	3-mo survival advantage conferred to patients receiving combined therapy (eg, surgery, brachytherapy & TMZ) compared with patients receiving TMZ rechallenge alone (P = .043)
Bekar et al,[63] 2012	Comparison of reoperation (n = 50) with no reoperation (n = 111) in patients who went on to receive adjuvant chemotherapy/RT in operative group	Reoperation at recurrence (P<.001), temporal vs parietal location associated with increased mortality (P = .01)
Bloch et al,[56] 2012	4-way comparison of resection status in initial surgery and on reoperation for recurrence of GBM: group 1: GTR, GTR (n = 31); group 2: GTR, STR (n = 21); group 3: STR, GTR (n = 26); group 4: STR, STR (n = 29)	Age (HR 1.03, P = .004), KPS at recurrence (HR 2.4, P = .02), EOR at reoperation (HR 0.62, P = .02) all significant in the Cox proportional hazards model STR/GTR mOS = 19.0 vs STR/STR mOS = 15.9 mo (P = .004)
Boiardi et al,[1] 2008	Comparison of salvage therapies at GBM recurrence: group 1: TMZ only (n = 161); group 2: surgery + TMZ (n = 50); group 3: surgery + TMZ + LR chemo (n = 65)	Second tumor debulking conferred a 36% decreased hazard of death (HR = 0.64; 0.46–0.89), local delivery of mitoxantrone reduced hazard of death to 50% (HR = 0.50; 0.38–0.68)
Chaichana et al,[44] 2013	Evaluation of the impact of multiple resections for GBM recurrence on survival in 4 groups of patients: group 1: initial operation (n = 354); group 2: reoperation (n = 168); group 3: reoperation × 2 (n = 41); group 4: reoperation × 3 (n = 15)	mOS = 6.8, 15.5, 22.4, & 26.6 mo for 1, 2, 3 & 4 resections, respectively (P<.05); 1 resection only = shortened survival (RR 3.400; P<.0001) vs ≥2 resections (RR 0.688; P = .0006)
Chen et al,[64] 2016	Comparison of patients who underwent reoperation and adjuvant therapy (n = 20) with those who receive adjuvant chemotherapy/RT (n = 45) for recurrent GBM	Age, KPS at recurrence, EOR for initial surgery, reoperation for recurrence; reoperation at GBM recurrence: mOS of 25.4 mo vs no reoperation at recurrence: 11.6 mo (P<.001); reoperation at GBM recurrence: rOS of 13.5 mo vs no reoperation at recurrence: 5.8 mo (P<.001)
Clarke et al,[8] 2011	NABTC trial pooled dataset of recurrent GBM: PFS at 6 mo & OS evaluated in patients who had reoperation for recurrence compared with those that did not within the context of a relatively homogenous clinical trial dataset	No difference in either PFS6 or OS in patients who underwent reoperation vs those who do not for tumor recurrence
De Bonis et al,[59] 2013	Comparison of combination salvage therapies in recurrent GBM group 1: surgery alone (n = 17); group 2: adjuvant chemotherapy alone (n = 24); group 3: surgery & adjuvant chemotherapy (n = 16); group 4: no intervention (n = 19)	Combination of reoperation and adjuvant chemotherapy improves survival (P = .01); KPS <70 were significantly at risk for death, HR 2.8 (P = .001)

(continued on next page)

Table 1
(continued)

Study/year	Study Description	Study Conclusions
Filippini et al,[50] 2008	Analysis of prognostic factors in a group of 676 consecutive patients with GBM, 544 treated on progression, 182 treated with reoperation	No effect of reoperation on survival, adjuvant chemotherapy (HR 0.61, $P = .001$) and radiation therapy (HR 0.89, $P = .04$); initial surgical resection in lieu of biopsy only in patients with good performance status regardless of age (HR 0.55, $P<.001$)
Franceschi et al,[51] 2015	Comparison of patients who underwent reoperation and adjuvant therapy (n = 102) with those who received adjuvant chemotherapy/RT (n = 130) for recurrent GBM	Reoperation did not affect survival ($P = .11$); age ($P = .001$), MGMT methylation ($P = .002$), and PFS6 ($P = .0001$) significantly correlated with improved OS
Gorlia et al,[7] 2012	EORTC phase I–II trial pooled dataset for patients with recurrent GBM treated with an experimental agent, a cytotoxic agent, or both independent of reoperation at recurrence; only 8% of patients had surgery for recurrence; prognostic factors evaluated including reoperation for GBM recurrence and predictive models calculated	ECOG >2 ($P = .009$), baseline steroids ($P = .02$), >1 target lesion ($P<.0001$), max diameter of the largest lesion (binary >42 mm, $P = .0003$)
Helseth et al,[43] 2010	Evaluation of the impact of multiple resections for GBM recurrence on survival in 4 groups of patients: group 1: initial operation (n = 451); group 2: reoperation (n = 55); group 3: reoperation × 2 (n = 8); group 4: reoperation × 3 (n = 2) and adjuvant therapies	Age >60 y (HR 1.02; $P<.01$), ECOG 3–4 at primary surgery (HR 2.13; $P<.001$), bilateral tumor representation (HR 2.31; $P<.001$), biopsy only at primary surgery (HR 2.72; $P<.01$), RT only without TMZ (HR 2.36; $P<.001$) on multivariate HR analysis; mOS = 18.4 mo for patients who underwent reoperation vs 8.6 mo for primary surgery only ($P<.001$)
Hong et al,[45] 2013	Comparison of more than one reoperation (n = 10) with one reoperation (n = 32) in patients who also had adjuvant therapy	PFS >3 mo as a significant independent prognostic factor ($P = .01$)
Kim et al,[52] 2015	Comparison of varying combination salvage therapies in recurrent GBM: group 1: GKS only (n = 29); group 2: TMZ only (n = 31); group 3: GKS + TMZ (n = 28); group 4: reoperation ± adjuvant chemotherapy or re-RT (n = 38); group 5: various chemotherapies, bevacizumab, methotrexate, and re-RT (n = 18)	Older age (HR 2.082, $P = .018$) & ECOG 2–4 (HR 1.624, $P = .027$) prognostic factors for a worse PFS ECOG 2–4 at progression (HR 1.924, $P = .003$), out of field, LMD at progression (HR 1.791, $P = .013$), PFS1 <9 mo (HR 1.992, $P = .002$) were poor prognostic factors for OS; GKS + TMZ good prognostic factor for PFS (HR 0.540, $P = .013$) & OS (HR 0.486, $P = .007$)
Ma et al,[53] 2009	Evaluation of multiple factors impacting survival in a review of 205 patients with GBM, 52 of which underwent reoperation	Age >55 y (RR 1.88; $P<.01$), KPS >80 at primary surgery (RR 2.449; $P<.01$) and poor tumor location (RR 2.335; $P<.01$), subtotal resection (RR 1.689; $P<.01$); reoperation not a predictive factor on multivariate analysis

(continued on next page)

Table 1
(continued)

Study/year	Study Description	Study Conclusions
Mandl et al,[60] 2008	Comparison of varying combination salvage therapies in recurrent GBM: group 1: conventional RT or SRS (n = 12); group 2: reoperation (n = 9); group 3: reoperation + conventional RT or SRS (n = 11)	Reoperation only for recurrent GBM associated with a shorter survival compared with RT/SRS alone and reoperation + RT/SRS Group 1: 28 wk; group 2: 13 wk; group 3: 34 wk; group 1 vs 2 (P = .025) & group 2 vs 3 (P = .0005) but not group 1 vs 3
McGirt et al,[65] 2008	3-way comparison of resection status (GTR, NTR, STR) in initial surgery (n = 451) and on reoperation for recurrence of GBM (n = 294)	NTR (37% risk reduction) & GTR (10% further risk reduction for a total of 47%) in relative risk of overall mortality compared with STR; age, KPS, EOR, postoperative TMZ all associated with enhanced survival after reoperation for recurrent GBM (P = .002– .009)
McNamara et al,[66] 2014	Evaluation of multiple factors impacting survival in a review of 107 patients undergoing reoperation for progressive/recurrent GBM	No chemo postreoperation portended worse survival (P<.001) on multivariate analysis; NLR >4 before reoperation a poor prognostic factor for postoperative survival in GBM; mOS after reoperation NLR <4 vs NLR >4 was 9.7 vs 5.9 mo, respectively (log-rank test P = .02)
Michaelson et al,[67] 2013	Review of varying combination salvage therapies in recurrent GBM: group 1: reoperation for recurrence (n = 74); group 2: bevacizumab/irinotecan (n = 85); group 3: TMZ alone (n = 12), a probability of survival model was designed	Reoperation (HR = 0.39; 95% CI, 0.25–0.60) and BEV/IRI (HR = 0.23; 95% CI, 0.15–0.34) at GBM recurrence improved rOS Combination therapy was superior to surgery alone (HR = 0.51; 95% CI, 0.31–0.83) but not BEV/IRI alone Age (P<.0001), ECOG 2 vs 0 score (P = .0015), corticosteroid therapy at RT/TMZ initiation (P<.0001) negatively impact mOS and rOS
Oppenlander et al,[58] 2014	Evaluation of the impact of extent of resection on survival in recurrent GBM (n = 170)	Age >67 y (P = .0001), KPS score (P = .001), and EOR >80% (P = .005) positive predictors of survival
Ortega et al,[31] 2016	Evaluation of the impact of multiple resections for GBM recurrence on survival in 3 groups of patients: group 1: reoperation (n = 83); group 2: reoperation × 2 (n = 94); group 3: reoperation × 3 (n = 25)	Older age at diagnosis only predictor of survival for patients with recurrent GBM (HR 1.34; 1.16–1.54, P<.0001); reoperation not predictive of survival
Park et al,[46] 2010	Review of prognostic factors influencing survival in patients with recurrent GBM (n = 34), creation of a prognostic scale, and then validated with a separate cohort (n = 109)	MSM score >2 (P<.001; HR 13.32), KPS score <80 (P<.001; HR 4.70), and tumor volume >50 cm^3 (P<.001; HR 7.63)
Park et al,[47] 2013	Review of prognostic factors influencing survival in patients with recurrent GBM (n = 55), creation of a prognostic scale, and then validated with a separate cohort (n = 96)	KPS of <70 (HR 0.395; 90% CI, 0.166–0.940; P<.078) & ependymal involvement (HR 0.411; 90% CI, 0.214–0.789; P<.025)

(continued on next page)

Table 1 *(continued)*		
Study/year	**Study Description**	**Study Conclusions**
Quick et al,[57] 2014	Evaluation of multiple factors impacting survival in a review of 40 patients who underwent reoperation for recurrent GBM with special attention paid to EOR	KPS, PFS, and complete tumor removal at second surgery independently associated with improved mOS (KPS, $P = .047$; PFS, $P = .019$; EOR, $P = .015$; Cox regression)
Ringel et al,[48] 2016	Evaluation of multiple resections for GBM recurrence on survival in 4 groups of patients: group 1: initial operation (n = 503); group 2: reoperation (n = 421); group 3: reoperation × 2 (n = 71); group 4: reoperation × 3 or more (n = 11)	Age at reoperation ($P = .017$), preoperative, and postoperative KPS ($P<.001$), EOR at first reoperation ($P<.001$) & chemotherapy after first reoperation ($P<.001$) all predictors of survival
Scorsetti et al,[68] 2015	Comparison of reoperation + adjuvant chemotherapy ± RT (n = 21) to chemotherapy only (n = 22)	Treatment modality associated with OS ($P = .01$) and PFS ($P = .004$); PFS12 65% for group 1 vs 22% for group 2 ($P<.01$; HR 2.5; CI 95% 1.21–5.28); PFS was 15 and 5 mo, respectively; 1-y OS was 69% for group 1% and 26% for group 2 ($P<.01$; HR 2.6; CI95% 1.24–5.45); median OS was 17 and 6 mo, respectively
Skeie et al,[20] 2012	3-way comparison of salvage therapies in recurrent GBM: group 1: GKS only (n = 32); group 2: reoperation (n = 26); group 3: reoperation + SRS (n = 19)	Actuarial local tumor control rates at 1, 3, 6, and 12 mo were 85.4%, 66.7%, 49.4%, and 25.0% after GKS treatment vs 76.0%, 36.0%, 16.0%, and 14.0% after reoperation GKS treatment, increased time to recurrence, adjuvant treatment, unifocal tumor, and tumor volume <20 mL favorable
Suchorska et al,[69] 2016	DIRECTOR trial dataset designed to explore TMZ rechallenge in GBM recurrence with post hoc analysis for extent of surgical resection: 3 surgical groups divided evenly; among the 2-arm chemotherapy study: group 1 complete resection of recurrent tumor; group 2: incomplete resection of recurrent tumor; group 3: no surgery All groups received TMZ rechallenge	On multivariate analysis: complete resection at recurrence improved survival (0.42 [0.21–0.85]; $P = .015$) In 12-mo survival rates analysis: 65% of patients with GTR were alive compared with 16.7% of those with incomplete resection ($P<.001$)
Sughrue et al,[54] 2015	Review of 104 patients undergoing reoperation for recurrent GBM (reoperation [n = 59], reoperation × 2 [n = 24], reoperation × 3–5 [n = 21]); factors predictive of PFS sought	PFS1 and PFS2 used to calculate a score RAI to test whether the time to progression of disease is predictive of tumor aggressivity after reoperation No evidence that one could predict aggressivity based on prior PFS
Tully et al,[55] 2016	Review of 204 patients with GBM, 49 of which were treated with surgery on recurrence: subgroup analysis excluding patients unlikely to be considered for reoperation carried out to combat confounding	Multivariable analysis showed reoperation (HR 0.646; 95% CI, 0.543–0.922; $P = .016$) and maximal initial adjuvant therapy (HR 0.337; 95% CI, 0.246–0.463; $P = .001$) associated with survival; finding of a survival benefit with reoperation was ameliorated by excluding unlikely surgical candidates

(continued on next page)

Table 1
(continued)

Study/year	Study Description	Study Conclusions
Woernle et al,[70] 2015	Comparison of reoperation (n = 40, group 1) with no reoperation (n = 58, group 2) in patients who went on to receive bevacizumab, TMZ, or lomustine: an amended NIH recurrent GBM scale conceived based on investigators' analysis	Age as the only predictor of reoperation at tumor progression (P = .012); alkylating agents (P = .004) and bevacizumab (P = .001) administration following reoperation led to longer OS; addition of age to the other 3 factors in the NIH recurrent GBM scale led to improved predictive value
Woodworth et al,[71] 2013	Histopathologic analysis with special attention to pseudoprogression (n = 17) during clinical data review of 59 patients reoperated on for presumed recurrent GBM	Decreased hazard of death: pseudoprogression histology (HR 0.6; P = .03), KPS >70 (HR 0.3; P = .03), initial GTR (0.6; P = .01) Portend poor survival after reoperation: DM (HR 2.3; P = .02), HTN (HR 2.1; P = .03), new neurologic deficit (HR 3.7; P = .01)
Yong et al,[72] 2014	Prospective longitudinal study evaluating prognostic factors for survival in a cohort of 97 patients who underwent surgery for recurrent GBM	Factors for larger postop tumor volume: eloquent location (OR = 16.00; P<.001) & larger preoperative tumor volume (P<.001); postoperative residual tumor volume associated with tumor regrowth rate on multiple logistic regression analysis (P = .003) Increased hazard of death: older age (HR 2.66; P = .003), lower KPS score (HR 6.08; P<.001), and progressively larger postoperative residual tumor volume (P<.001)

Abbreviations: BEV/IRI, Bevacizumab/Irinotecan; CI, confidence interval; DM, diabetes mellitus; EOR, extent of resection; EORTC, European Organization for Research and Treatment of Cancer; GKS, gamma knife radiosurgery; GTR, gross total resection; HDR, High dose rate as in high dose rate brachytherapy; HR, hazard ratio; HTN, hypertension; KPS, Karnofsky performance scale; LR, Log-rank test; LMD, leptomeningeal disease; MGMT, O(6)-methylguanine-DNA methyltransferase; MSM, Motor-Speech-Middle cerebral artery score; NABTC, North American Brain Tumor Consortium; NIH, National Institutes of Health; NLR, neutrophil/lymphocyte ratio; NTR, Near total resection; OR, odds ratio; RAI, relative aggressivity index; RR, risk ratio; SRS, Stereotactic radiosurgery; STR, subtotal resection.

radiologically confirmed recurrence via either MacDonald's or Response Assessment in Neuro-Oncology (RANO) criteria. Many, though not all, studies required adjuvant therapy with TMZ chemoradiotherapy after initial diagnosis. Common exclusion criteria include infratentorial or thalamic location, multifocal or bihemispheric tumor status, known secondary GBM status, poor PS (KPS <50–60, ECOG >3–4), incomplete medical records, and histology suggestive of pseudoprogression.

Indications for Surgery

Indications for surgery included obvious radiographic progression on surveillance imaging in accordance with either the MacDonald or RANO criteria and clinical decline including paresis or altered mental status as a manifestation of elevated intracranial pressure, mass effect, or seizures. Recommendation from a multidisciplinary tumor board was listed as an indication to proceed with reoperation, as were patients with good PS and focal disease amenable to complete resection and (see **Table 4**).

Survival Following Reoperation for Recurrent or Progressive Glioblastoma Multiforme

The incorporation of the regimen of concomitant chemoradiotherapy with TMZ followed by adjuvant TMZ, as described by Roger Stupp and colleagues[27] and others[2,28,29] in the early twenty-first century, has led to improved survival for patients diagnosed with GBM. Per recent clinical trial data and specialized center reports, it is more frequently the case that patients are achieving median survival in the 20-month range.[3,30,31] These developments underscore

Table 2
Study author, year, and design for original articles addressing reoperation and extent of resection

Design	Study/Year	Benefit of Surgery at Recurrence	EOR Benefit at Recurrence
Prospective study or prospectively collected data	Archavalis et al,[62] 2014	Yes	—
	Michaelson et al,[67] 2013	Yes	No
	Suchorska et al,[69] 2016	Yes	Yes
	Yong et al,[72] 2014	Yes	Yes
	Clarke et al,[8] 2011	No	—
	Gorlia et al,[7] 2012	No	—
Retrospective studies	Bekar et al,[63] 2012	Yes	—
	Boiardi et al,[1] 2008	Yes	Yes
	Bloch et al,[56] 2012	Yes	Yes
	Chen et al,[64] 2016	Yes	No
	Chaichana et al,[44] 2013	Yes	—
	De Bonis et al,[59] 2013	Yes	No
	Helseth et al,[43] 2010	Yes	—
	Hong et al,[45] 2013	Yes	No
	Mandl et al,[60] 2008	Yes	—
	McGirt et al,[38] 2009	Yes	Yes
	McNamara et al,[66] 2014	Yes	No
	Oppenlander et al,[58] 2014	Yes	Yes
	Quick et al,[57] 2014	Yes	Yes
	Ringel et al,[48] 2016	Yes	Yes
	Scorsetti et al,[68] 2015	Yes	—
	Woernle et al,[70] 2015	Yes	—
	Filippini et al,[50] 2008	No	—
	Franceschi et al,[51] 2015	No	—
	Kim et al,[52] 2015	No	No
	Ma et al,[53] 2009	No	Yes
	Ortega et al,[31] 2016	No	Yes
	Skeie et al,[20] 2012	No	—
	Sughrue et al,[54] 2015	No	—
	Tully et al,[55] 2016	No	—
	Park et al,[46] 2010	—	—
	Park et al,[47] 2013	—	—
	Woodworth et al,[71] 2013	—	—

continued progress being made in the field over the past 2 decades.

As nonsurgical adjunctive therapies advance so too is our understanding of the impact of surgery on survival in both newly diagnosed and recurrent GBM. Multiple studies have demonstrated a survival benefit in maximizing the EOR in newly diagnosed GBM.[5,32–37] Despite being largely predicated on class II to III evidence, it has become generally accepted that less residual tumor equates to longer PFS and higher overall survival, if preservation of neurologic function is maintained.[38–41] There is enough granularity in the analysis of EOR data in newly diagnosed GBM to quantify the survival benefit of a gross total resection (GTR) at approximately 3.5 to 5.0 months.[39,40]

Unfortunately, the role of reoperation in recurrent or progressive disease is less clear despite some estimates indicating that reoperation may provide a similar survival benefit of 3 to 5 months.[10] The mOS reported in the literature after disease

Table 3
Complications

Study/Year	Complications
Archavalis et al,[62] 2014	18% rate of surgical complications (eg, infection, CSF leak, grade 3/4 hemorrhage) 4 of 66 patients radiation necrosis 33% grade 3/4 thrombocytopenia & leukopenia
Boiardi et al,[1] 2008	Surgical complications: 6.0% transient focal deficit, 9.0% hemorrhage, 12.3% reservoir infection, 9.0% abscess; rates of chemo-toxicity: 16.5% grade 3/4 leukopenia and 18.1% grade 3/4 thrombocytopenia
Chaichana et al,[44] 2013	No difference between patients with 1 or more reoperations
De Bonis et al,[59] 2013	Major surgical morbidity 48% (16 of 33 patients)
Helseth et al,[43] 2010	Mortality at first (3.3%), second (3.1%), third (0.0%), and fourth (0.0%) surgeries
Mandl et al,[60] 2008	15% permanent neurologic morbidity, 5% mortality
Oppenlander et al,[58] 2014	7-d postoperative rate of deterioration in NIHSS >1: For >80.0% resection (39.1%) & >90.0% resection (45.8%) vs <80.0% resection (16.7%) & <90.0% resection (25.4%) (P = .0049); 15.0% & 9.0% of patients developed new or worsened neurologic deficits after surgery, respectively
Quick et al,[57] 2014	Complications in 19.9% of patients, 15.0% new or worsened neurologic deficit, 7.5% wound revision for CSF leak or infection
Ringel et al,[58] 2016	Increase with subsequent surgery: Initial surgery 5% non-neurological complications, 7% transient, and 5% permanent neurologic deficits compared with 7% non-neurological complications, 9% transient, and 8% permanent neurologic deficits
Scorsetti et al,[68] 2015	No acute worsening of neurologic function or return to the operating room, no perioperative mortality, grade 1/2 hematologic toxicity found in 8 (20%) patients
Skeie et al,[20] 2012	26.7% complication rate; 20.0% worsened neurologically, one death due to postoperative hemorrhage; 9.8% rate of complication after SRS
Suchorska et al,[69] 2016	Excluded patients with serious postoperative complications
Sughrue et al,[54] 2015	18% of reoperated patients had a new or worsened motor examination: 4.8% speech disturbance, 2.9% wound infection (all after third craniotomy, 2 of 3 on bevacizumab), 1.9% CSF leak; no difference in any complication between second and 3–6 operations groups
Tully et al,[55] 2016	17.2% complication at initial surgery
Woernle et al,[70] 2015	Initial surgery 11 of 98 or 11.2% patients with a complication (unspecified); no data available for reoperated patients
Yong et al,[72] 2014	Overall complication rate = 7.2%

Abbreviations: CSF, cerebrospinal fluid; NIHSS, National Institutes of Health Stroke Scale.

recurrence is 5.8 to 8.1 months.[1,9] Barbagallo and colleagues[10] report median survival following reoperation for recurrent GBM at 3 to 13 months. Of the 33 studies evaluated in this review, 20 noted a survival benefit of reoperation and 10 did not (see **Table 2**). The average median survival following reoperation in the present review was found to be 9.9 months, which is in accordance with other estimates in the literature.[10]

Barker and colleagues[11] reviewed prospectively collected clinical trial data to evaluate the survival and functional impact of reoperation for recurrent GBM in 1998. Forty-six of 301 patients underwent reoperation within 2 years of their initial diagnosis, and the median survival following resection was 9 months. Higher preoperative KPS scores and reoperation predicted longer overall survival, but the investigators determined that this was at least partially due to selection bias. High-quality survival (KPS >70) was 18 weeks.

Stark and colleagues[42] retrospectively evaluated 72 of 267 patients who had initial surgery for GBM diagnosis and then went on to have reoperation at the time of disease recurrence. The mOS was 11.7 months. Age less than 61 years, KPS

Table 4
Indications for reoperation

Study/Year	Surgical Indication
Boiardi et al,[1] 2008	Recurrence judged resectable without risk of neurologic deficit
Chen et al,[64] 2016	Progression on imaging, focal neurologic deficit, ICP, mass effect, altered consciousness, or uncontrolled seizures
Clarke et al,[8] 2011	Imaging recurrence
Gorlia et al,[7] 2012	Radiographic recurrence (Macdonald criteria) indication for treatment
Helseth et al,[43] 2010	Neurologic deficit, mass effect, ICP, seizures, MRI recurrence
Mandl et al,[60] 2008	KPS >70, no multifocal disease, lesion amenable to meaningful resection
Oppenlander et al,[58] 2014	Imaging evidence of recurrence
Ortega et al,[31] 2016	Radiographic progression
Park et al,[46] 2010	Radiographic progression
Park et al,[47] 2013	Radiographic progression (Macdonald criteria)
Quick et al,[57] 2014	Multidisciplinary tumor board recommendation, amenable to near total resection KPS >60
Suchorska et al,[69] 2016	Multidisciplinary tumor board recommendation
Sughrue et al,[54] 2015	Radiographic progression (RANO)
Tully et al,[55] 2016	Radiographic or clinical progression & imaging review
Woodworth et al,[71] 2013	Clinical worsening in the setting of new imaging findings, multidisciplinary tumor board, benefit from debulking/tissue diagnosis

Abbreviations: ICP, intracranial pressure; KPS, Karnofsky performance scale; RANO, Response Assessment in Neuro-Oncology.

greater than 70, radiotherapy dose (RT) greater than 54 Gy, chemotherapy, GTR, and reoperation were all associated with prolonged survival.

Helseth and colleagues[43] retrospectively reviewed a single institution, multicenter, prospectively collected database for analysis of 516 consecutive patients who underwent initial surgery for GBM. Repeat surgery was carried out in 65 patients. The median time between first and second surgery was 7 months; most, although not all, of the patients had TMZ therapy. For those patients undergoing repeat operations, the mOS was significantly longer using Kaplan-Meier analysis (18.4 vs 8.6 months, $P<.001$). Poor prognostic factors included age greater than 60 years, ECOG greater than 2, bilateral tumor, biopsy rather than resection, and absence of TMZ therapy.[43]

More recently, articles have begun to look at the impact of multiple resections on survival.[44,45] Chaichana and colleagues[44] conducted a single-center chart review of 354 patients who underwent initial surgery for diagnosis, 168 patients of whom had a second surgery at GBM recurrence. Forty-one more patients had a third surgery, and 15 patients further had 4 resections. The median survival of the entire cohort was 10.7 months. After controlling for known positive prognostic factors (age, neurologic status, periventricular location,

EOR, and adjuvant therapy) with a multivariate analysis and case-control analysis, the investigators observed a statistically significant dose-response effect of reoperation on survival with mOS for 1, 2, 3, or 4 resections reported as 6.8, 15.5, 22.4, and 26.6 months, respectively.

In 2010, Park and colleagues[46] fashioned the National Institutes of Health (NIH) Recurrent GBM Scale from retrospective analysis of clinical and radiographic factors associated with decreased survival in a cohort of patients treated at the NIH. The scale was subsequently validated in a contemporary cohort at the Brigham and Women's Hospital and uses 3 criteria with 1 point allocated for each criterion: the Motor-Speech-Middle cerebral artery score, KPS less than 80, and tumor volume greater than 50 mL. The results are additive with a range of 0 to 3 (0 = good, mOS 10.8 months; 1–2 = intermediate, mOS 4.5 months; and 3 = poor, mOS 1 month).

Using similar methodology an amended version of the scale was published in 2013 with only 2 clinical factors in an effort to improve practicality: KPS (0 for KPS $\geq$70 and 1 for KPS <70) and ependymal involvement (0 for no enhancement of ventricular wall on MRI and 1 for enhancement). The results are additive with a range of 0 to 2 (0 = good, mOS 18 months; 1 = intermediate, mOS 10 months; and 2 = poor, mOS 4 months).[47]

Table 5
Survival in reoperated GBM

Study/Year	mOS	rOS	PFS	PFS1
Archavalis et al,[62] 2014	Group 1: 7.8 mo group 2: 8.2 mo, group 3: 8.0 mo Historical control (ddTMZ): 5 months* statistically significant via LR test	Group 1: 20 mo, group 2: 21 mo, group 3: 20.5 Historical control (dose dense TMZ): 14 mo	—	—
Bekar et al,[63] 2012	26.7 mo in reoperative group vs 12.2 mo in nonreoperative group*; statistical significance reached via regression analysis	—	—	—
Bloch et al,[56] 2012	Group 1: GTR, GTR = 20.4 mo; group 2: GTR, STR = 18.4 mo; group 3: STR, GTR = 19.0 mo; group 4: STR, STR = 15.9 mo* Statistical significance reached via KM LR test only for group 3 vs group 4	Group 1: GTR, GTR = 11.5 mo; group 2: GTR, STR = 8.5 mo; group 3: STR, GTR = 16.7 mo; group 4: STR, STR = 7.4 mo* Statistical significance reached via KM LR test only for group 3 vs group 4	GTR (mean 11.3 mo) vs STR (mean 6.7 mo, P = .009)	—
Boiardi et al,[1] 2008	—	Group 1: 5 mo, group 2: 8 mo, group 3: surgery + TMZ + LR chemo 11 mo	—	Group 1: 39.4%, group 2: 64.0%, group 3: 70.7% survival at 6 mo
Chaichana et al,[44] 2013	mOS = 6.8, 15.5, 22.4, & 26.6 mo for 1, 2, 3, & 4 resections, respectively (P<.05)	—	—	—
Chen et al,[64] 2016	Group 1: 25.4 mo compared with group 2: 11.6 mo	Reoperation at GBM recurrence: 13.5 mo vs 5.8 mo for no reoperation (P<.001)	—	—
Clarke et al,[8] 2011	8.275 mo	8.275 mo	—	2.3 mo
De Bonis et al,[59] 2013	—	Group 1: 6 mo, group 2: 8 mo, group 3: 14 mo,* group 4: 5 mo (P = .01)	—	—
Filippini et al,[50] 2008	Effect of initial surgical resection vs biopsy only = 8-mo mOS advantage mOS was 13.6 mo for the entire cohort of patients with GBM	6.1 mo Reoperation did not effect survival time	—	—

Study				
Franceschi et al,[51] 2015	mOS = 25.8 mo in the reoperated group vs 18.6 mo in the chemotherapy-alone group In the multivariate analysis no difference by reoperation status found	9.6 mo in the reoperation group vs 7.5 mo in the chemotherapy only group (P = .3)	—	—
Gorlia et al,[7] 2012	—	6.2 mo for all patients with GBM, PFS at 1 y = 22.1%	—	1.8 mo, PFS6 of 14.7%
Helseth et al,[43] 2010	mOS for reoperation = 18.4 mo vs 8.6 mo for primary surgery only (P<.001) mOS for all patients with recurrent GBM = 9.9 mo	—	7.0 mo (time to reoperation)	—
Hong et al,[45] 2013	mOS >1 reoperation = 26 mo vs 16 mo for 1 reoperation only (P = .052) Multiple reoperation group 2-y (58%) & 3-y (31%) survival rates vs 29.0% & 12.4% at 2 y and 3 y, respectively, for those undergoing 1 reoperation only (P = .036, P = .032)	—	—	—
Kim et al,[52] 2015	For the entire cohort of patients with recurrent GBM mOS = 18.7	Group 1: 9.2 mo, group 2: 5.6 mo, group 3: 15.5 mo, group 4: 13.2 mo, group 5: 8.0 mo rOS from the beginning of salvage treatment = 9.9 mo for all groups	8.8 mo	Group 1: 3.6 mo, group 2: 2.3 mo, group 3: 6.0 mo, group 4: 4.3 mo, group 5: 2.6 mo Median PFS from salvage treatment = 3.9 mo for all groups
Ma et al,[53] 2009	12 mo for all GBM, mOS with postoperative RT = OS 15.0 mo vs 8.0 mo without Radical surgery mOS = 14.0 mo vs 8.0 mo for partial surgery at primary surgery (P = .02) No survival advantage for reoperation with GBM recurrence	—	—	—

(continued on next page)

Table 5
(continued)

Study/Year	mOS	rOS	PFS	PFS1
Mandl et al,[60] 2008	mOS of all recurrent patients = 62 wk	Group 1: 28 wk, group 2: 13 wk, group 3: 34 wk; statistical significance comparison of group 1 vs 2 (P = .025) & group 2 vs 3 (P = .0005) but not group 1 vs 3	—	—
McGirt et al,[38] 2009	mOS for GTR (13 mo), NTR (11 mo), and STR (8 mo) Statistical significance reached between all comparisons (P = .002–.04)	mOS for GTR (11 mo), NTR (9 mo), and STR (5 mo) Statistical significance reached between all comparisons (P = .002–.048)	—	—
McNamara et al,[66] 2014	Reoperation mOS = 20.9 mo vs 9.9 mo in primary surgery only (P = .001) mOS after reoperation in patients with NLR <4 vs NLR >4 was 9.7 vs 5.9 mo (P = .02)	Following reoperation for recurrent GBM when PFS was <12 mo, 12–24 mo, or >24 mo, mOS was 7.2, 7.0, and 6.3 mo, respectively (P = .6)	7.8 mo	—
Michaelson et al,[67] 2013	mOS for entire cohort = 14.3 mo	Following tumor recurrence, mOS = 5.9 mo	8.0 mo	—
Oppenlander et al,[58] 2014	mOS reoperation = 19.0 mo, 80% EOR at reoperation = 19.2-mo median survival EOR ≥81% = 20-mo mOS, EOR of ≥97% = 30.0-mo mOS Continued mOS improvement seen within the 95%–100% range (P<.001)	—	—	5.2 mo
Ortega et al,[31] 2016	mOS for entire cohort = 23.6 mo; group 1: 21.1 mo, group 2: 25.5 mo, group 3: 29.0 mo (P = .03) Not significant in the confounder-adjusted multivariate model	—	7.0 mo	—

Study	Findings			
Park et al,[46] 2010	Additive scale (range, 0–3 points), 3 variables distinguishes mOS after reoperation Good (0 points, 10.8 mo), intermediate (1–2 points, 4.5 mo), and poor (3 points, 1.0 mo) NIH recurrent GBM scale scores (P<.001)	7.4 mo		—
Park et al,[47] 2013	Additive scale (range, 0–2 points) 2 variables distinguishes mOS after reoperation Good (0 points, 18.0 mo), intermediate (1 point, 10.0 mo; P<.006) Poor (2 points, 4.0 mo; P<.000) status (P<.001)	10.0 mo	12.0 mo (time to reoperation)	—
Quick et al,[57] 2014	Recurrent GBM cohort treated with reoperation mOS = 21.7 mo For complete resection mOS = 26.0 mo vs 18.8 mo incomplete resection (P = .015)	13.5 mo	10.2 mo	13.0 mo
Ringel et al,[58] 2016	Group 1: 25.0 mo, group 2: 22.7 mo, group 3: 29.3 mo, group 4: 34.3 mo	11.9 mo	9.1 mo	7.0 mo
Scorsetti et al,[68] 2015	For reoperation, chemotherapy ± RT (group 1), mOS = 17 mo vs 6 mo for chemotherapy-only (group 2) Group 1 survival rates: 69% and 29% at 1 and 2 y vs group 2: 26% and 0% (P<.01; HR 2.6)	11.0 mo	13.0 mo	8.0 mo
Skeie et al,[20] 2012	Whole cohort of recurrent GBM = 17 mo Group 1: 19 mo, group 2: 16 mo (P = .021, HR 1.8)	12.0 mo for the 51 patients receiving GKS (group 1 + group 3) vs 6 mo in patients undergoing reoperation only (P = .001, HR 2.4)		6 mo in those patients undergoing GKS (95% CI: 2.86–9.14) vs 2 mo (95% CI: 0.61–3.39) after resection (P = .009, × 2 = 9.4)

(continued on next page)

Table 5
(continued)

Study/Year	mOS	rOS	PFS	PFS1
Suchorska et al,[69] 2016	—	11.4 mo (95% CI: 8.4–12.3) reoperation vs 9.8 mo (95% CI: 6.6–15.1) in patients who did not undergo surgery ($P = .633$) Complete resection at reoperation vs incomplete resection rOS = 12.9 vs 6.5 mo ($P<.001$)	—	In patients who underwent complete resection/reoperation for GBM recurrence PFS2 = 3.5 mo No reoperation = 1.87 mo ($P = .05$)
Sughrue et al,[54] 2015	—	—	—	Median PFS from reoperation = 7.8 mo, from second reoperation = 6.0 mo 3–5 reoperations = 4.8 mo (Kaplan-Meier analysis = no significant difference)
Tully et al,[55] 2016	mOS for all patients = 12 mo (95% CI, 10.1–13.8) Reoperation mOS = 20.1 mo vs 9.0 mo without surgery ($P = .001$) Selecting out posterior fossa location, aged >80 y, ECOG ≥2, no survival advantage for reoperation on recurrent GBM was found (8.4 vs 8.9, $P = .158$)	7.6 mo	7.3 mo	—

Woernle et al,[70] 2015	Group 1: 18.86 mo vs group 2: 14.81 mo (P = .001)	8.33 mo (SD 1.01; 95% CI 5.93–13.1) in the intermediate category; 13.93 mo (SD 1.23; lower 95% CI 11.48) in the good category	—
Woodworth et al,[71] 2013	Entire cohort of patients with presumed recurrent GBM = 20-mo mOS	8.0 mo, however, patients found to have pseudoprogression (n = 17) lived nearly twice as long as patients with histopathologic diagnosis of recurrent GBM (n = 42, P = .03)	9.3 mo (time to reoperation)
Yong et al,[72] 2014	—	12.4 mo	—

Abbreviations: CI, confidence interval; ddTMZ, dose-dense temozolomide; ECOG, Eastern Cooperative Oncology Group; GTR, gross total resection; HR, hazard ratio; KM, Kaplan-Meier; LR, Log-rank test; NIH, National Institutes of Health; NLR, neutrophil/lymphocyte ratio; STR, subtotal resection.

* Statistical significance in a specific subgroup or analysis and is indicated in the table.

This year some of the largest cohorts of recurrent GBM to date have been published.[31,48,49] Ringel and colleagues examined 421, 71, and 11 patients who underwent reoperation once, twice, and more than 3 times, respectively. The mOS for the entire cohort was 25.0 months. Subsequent mOS for first, second, third, and fourth reoperations are 22.7 (95% confidence interval [CI] 21.2–26.2), 29.3 (95% CI 24.9–40.6), 34.3 (95% CI 34.3, not available [n.a]), and 26.4 months (24.7, n.a), respectively. Age at reoperation (P = .017), preoperative, and postoperative KPS (P<.001), EOR at the first reoperation (P<.001), and chemotherapy after first reoperation (P<.001) were all found to be predictors of survival on multivariate analysis, but reoperation was not. This theme of no survival advantage to reoperation was repeated 9 more times for articles included in the present review.[7,8,20,31,50–55]

Extent of resection

Multiple studies have evaluated the benefit of an increased EOR on survival at the time of the first surgery.[5,34–38] It seems that a 3.5- to 5.5-month survival benefit is imparted on gross total removal of the contrast-enhancing tumor on diagnosis. It is less clear if such an advantage is conferred again during reoperation for recurrence. Of the data included in the present review, 16 studies examined EOR as a factor associated with enhanced survival, 10 of which were affirmed (see **Table 2**). Boiardi and colleagues[1] used a cutoff of 3 cm maximal diameter to describe the size of the resection cavity plus residual contrast-enhancing tumor after reoperation. For patients with a resection cavity/residual tumor volume of 3 cm or less mOS was 16.2 months and for those 3 cm or greater mOS was 9.0 months (P<.001).

Bloch and colleagues[56] evaluated 107 patients with multiple resections and conducted a 4-way group analysis dependent on one of 4 possible resection statuses: GTR or subtotal resection (STR) at initial surgery followed by GTR or STR at subsequent surgery. These surgical resection status combinations yield 4 possible EOR groups: GTR/GTR, GTR/STR, STR/GTR, or STR/STR. Thirty-one patients underwent GTR/GTR, 21 had GTR/STR, 26 had STR/GTR, and 29 had STR/STR. Median actuarial survival for GTR/GTR = 20.4 months, GTR/STR = 18.4 months, STR/GTR = 19.0 months, and in STR/STR = 15.9 months (statistically significant survival advantage of STR/GTR over STR/STR, P = .004). Survival was similar between patients with GTR at initial surgery and in patients who had STR at initial surgery provided those initial STR patients underwent GTR at reoperation (19.1 vs 18.7 months).[56,57] As has been discussed previously, these findings suggest that the survival advantage rendered with complete resection at initial surgery may be salvaged at the time of disease recurrence.[57]

Oppenlander and colleagues[58] found a survival advantage when reoperation for recurrent GBM resulted in at least 80% resection.[5] The mOS for the entire cohort was 19.0 months. Greater than 81% resection yielded a 20-month mOS, and more than 97% resection was associated with a 30-month median survival on Kaplan-Meier analysis. Multivariate analysis identified EOR, age, and KPS as independent predictors of survival.

Progression-free survival

Surprisingly, PFS as a predictive factor of improved overall survival was only identified on multivariate analysis in 4 studies in the present review.[45,48,51,57] Sughrue and colleagues[54] designed a study to determine if the PFS period between 2 reoperations could be used to predict tumor behavior and, thus, more accurately predict patient survival. (PFS1 = time from initial surgery to reoperation number 1 and PFS2 = time from reoperation number 1 to reoperation number 2). The relationship PFS1/PFS2 describes the relative aggressivity index (RAI). RAI values closer to 2 indicate more aggressive disease and values closer to 0.5 represent less aggressive disease. After review of 59, 24, and 21 patients who underwent 1, 2, and 3 to 5 reoperations, respectively, the investigators concluded "previous PFS is entirely unable to predict the PFS that another surgery will provide the patient."[54]

Complications

The goal of surgical intervention for patients with a GBM at any point during the disease course is safe, maximal cytoreduction. Surgical intervention is not without risk owing to the highly infiltrative nature of the disease, the frequent incidence of these tumors in eloquent, deep-seated, or periventricular locations and the older comorbid status of patients who frequently have this disease. Complication rates quoted in the literature vary from 13% to 69% morbidity and from 0% to 11% mortality.[10] Sixteen investigators reported complication data yielding an approximate estimated complication rate of 18.9% (see **Table 3**).

In a recent group of highly selected patients with recurrent GBM treated in a neurosurgical department with the capacity to enroll patients in clinical trials and use 5-aminolevulinic acid–guided microsurgery and neuronavigational techniques, 16 of 33 patients had considerable operative morbidity.[59] According to De Bonis and colleagues,[59] in many cases these patients were unable to proceed to adjuvant therapy. As a possible consequence, there was no difference in survival between patients undergoing reoperation at recurrence without adjuvant therapy and those patients who received no treatment at all at recurrence, underscoring the importance of morbidity-free surgery on survival and emphasizing the importance of judicious decision-making for our patients. The risk of a complication has been estimated in surgery for newly diagnosed GBM.[38,40,41] Data like these suggest the risk of getting worse after surgery may have a similar effect on survival in recurrent GBM as well. Forty percent of patients in the study by Mandl and colleagues[60] had a postoperative decrement in KPS. Three of 20 patients developed a permanent neurologic morbidity, and there was 1 mortality in 20 reoperations, further underscoring the risk involved in surgery for recurrent disease. A large, multicenter retrospective series of more than 400 patients undergoing reoperation for recurrent disease demonstrates a slight increase in the rate of non-neurologic complications and neurologic deficits when comparing initial surgery for diagnosis with first reoperation for recurrent disease (5% non-neurological complications, 7% transient, and 5% permanent neurologic deficits compared with 7% non-neurological complications, 9% transient, and 8% permanent neurologic deficits).[48]

Bias

Bias in studies evaluating surgery for patients with recurrent GBM is a major confounder and can prevent accurate assessment of results. At a minimum there are several biases in play within the present review and its included studies. First, narrowing inclusion criteria to compensate for study heterogeneity can inadvertently restrict results to those being reported in a specific way, potentially leading to missed data and incorrect conclusions.[61] Second, in a comprehensive review there is bound to be publication bias, as negative studies are less often published and the gray literature and scientific meeting abstracts are not often searched. Thirdly, recall bias is inherent to any retrospective study. Perhaps most importantly, the selection bias that is driven by complex surgical decision-making on the parts of surgeons and patients continue to play the role of confounder.

Tully and colleagues[55] point out that in studies evaluating the survival benefit of reoperation there is often a comparison group that does not undergo reoperation. This nonoperative comparison group typically has a disproportionate number of patients who would never actually be considered as surgical candidates, thereby biasing the results in favor of reoperation inasmuch as the two groups are not balanced for all factors that may positively influence outcome after surgery. Tully and colleagues[55] explore this potential bias by first evaluating 2 cohorts of patients with recurrent GBM, those who underwent reoperation and those who did not. A significant difference in survival between the cohorts was demonstrated, and both univariate and multivariate analyses clearly demonstrated an advantage in the reoperation cohort. On subsequent subgroup analysis, the selecting out of patients with factors unlikely to be associated with candidates for reoperation (eg, posterior fossa location, aged >70 years, ECOG ≥2), the survival advantage thought to be imparted by reoperation for recurrence disappeared.

SUMMARY

Invariably, primary and review articles addressing GBM recurrence offer a disclaimer avowing the fact that the largely retrospective nature of the data and heterogeneity of surgical decision-making are major limitations when drawing conclusions from the literature. Undoubtedly this is true, but there are certainly conclusions that can be drawn from the depth of work and wealth of experience that has been published. Namely, that the decision to operate on recurrence is a significant one that should be made with perhaps even more thoughtfulness than in patients presenting for initial diagnosis. The focus should remain on those prognostic factors that are consistently verified across the literature regardless of its current limitations (see **Table 1**). Accordingly, most studies have confirmed a role for performance status, age, focal versus multifocal disease, favorable disease location, lower preoperative tumor size, and greater likelihood of complete resection and safe surgery as predictors of improved survival.

ACKNOWLEDGMENTS

The authors would like to thank Antonio P. DeRosa, MLIS, AHIP, of Memorial Sloan Kettering Cancer Center Library Sciences for his assistance with our literature search.

REFERENCES

1. Boiardi A, Silvani A, Eoli M, et al. Treatment of recurrent glioblastoma: can local delivery of mitoxantrone improve survival? J Neurooncol 2008;88(1):105–13.
2. Ostrom QT, Gittleman H, Fulop J, et al. CBTRUS statistical report: primary brain and central nervous system tumors diagnosed in the United States in 2008-2012. Neuro Oncol 2015;17(Suppl 4):iv1–62.

3. Sampson JH. Alternating electric fields for the treatment of glioblastoma. JAMA 2015;314(23):2511–3.

4. Elder JB, Chiocca EA. Editorial: glioblastoma multiforme and laser interstitial thermal therapy. J Neurosurg 2013;118(6):1199–201.

5. Sanai N, Polley M-Y, McDermott MW, et al. An extent of resection threshold for newly diagnosed glioblastomas. J Neurosurg 2011;115(1):3–8.

6. Mann BS. Overall survival benefit from surgical resection in treatment of recurrent glioblastoma. Ann Oncol 2014;25(9):1866–7.

7. Gorlia T, Stupp R, Brandes AA, et al. New prognostic factors and calculators for outcome prediction in patients with recurrent glioblastoma: a pooled analysis of EORTC Brain Tumour Group phase I and II clinical trials. Eur J Cancer 2012;48(8):1176–84.

8. Clarke JL, Ennis MM, Yung WKA, et al. Is surgery at progression a prognostic marker for improved 6-month progression-free survival or overall survival for patients with recurrent glioblastoma? Neuro Oncol 2011;13(10):1118–24.

9. Weller M, Cloughesy T, Perry JR, et al. Standards of care for treatment of recurrent glioblastoma–are we there yet? Neuro Oncol 2013;15(1):4–27.

10. Barbagallo GMV, Jenkinson MD, Brodbelt AR. "Recurrent" glioblastoma multiforme, when should we reoperate? Br J Neurosurg 2008;22(3):452–5.

11. Barker FG 2nd, Chang SM, Gutin PH, et al. Survival and functional status after resection of recurrent glioblastoma multiforme. Neurosurgery 1998;42(4):709–20 [discussion: 720–3].

12. Chang SM, Parney IF, McDermott M, et al. Perioperative complications and neurological outcomes of first and second craniotomies among patients enrolled in the Glioma Outcome Project. J Neurosurg 2003;98(6):1175–81.

13. Ryken TC, Frankel B, Julien T, et al. Surgical management of newly diagnosed glioblastoma in adults: role of cytoreductive surgery. J Neurooncol 2008;89(3):271–86.

14. Ammirati M, Vick N, Liao YL, et al. Effect of the extent of surgical resection on survival and quality of life in patients with supratentorial glioblastomas and anaplastic astrocytomas. Neurosurgery 1987;21(2):201–6.

15. Soults CB, Canute GS, Ryken TC. Evidence-based review of the role of reoperation in the management of malignant glioma. Neurosurg Focus 1998;4(6):e11.

16. Hervey-Jumper SL, Berger MS. Reoperation for recurrent high-grade glioma: a current perspective of the literature. Neurosurgery 2014;75(5):491–9.

17. Chowdhary SA, Ryken T, Newton HB. Survival outcomes and safety of carmustine wafers in the treatment of high-grade gliomas: a meta-analysis. J Neurooncol 2015;122(2):367–82.

18. Dirks P, Bernstein M, Muller PJ, et al. The value of reoperation for recurrent glioblastoma. Can J Surg 1993;36(3):271–5.

19. Strömblad LG, Anderson H, Malmström P, et al. Reoperation for malignant astrocytomas: personal experience and a review of the literature. Br J Neurosurg 1993;7(6):623–33.

20. Skeie BS, Enger PO, Brogger J, et al. Gamma knife surgery versus reoperation for recurrent glioblastoma multiforme. World Neurosurg 2012;78(6):658–69.

21. Salcman M, Kaplan RS, Ducker TB, et al. Effect of age and reoperation on survival in the combined modality treatment of malignant astrocytoma. Neurosurgery 1982;10(4):454–63.

22. Durmaz R, Erken S, Arslantaş A, et al. Management of glioblastoma multiforme: with special reference to recurrence. Clin Neurol Neurosurg 1997;99(2):117–23.

23. Rostomily RC, Spence AM, Duong D, et al. Multimodality management of recurrent adult malignant gliomas: results of a phase II multiagent chemotherapy study and analysis of cytoreductive surgery. Neurosurgery 1994;35(3):378–88 [discussion: 388].

24. Weller M, Wick W. Neuro-oncology in 2013: Improving outcome in newly diagnosed malignant glioma. Nat Rev Neurol 2014;10(2):68–70.

25. Ryken TC, Kalkanis SN, Buatti JM, et al. The role of cytoreductive surgery in the management of progressive glioblastoma: a systematic review and evidence-based clinical practice guideline. J Neurooncol 2014;118(3):479–88.

26. Montemurro N, Perrini P, Blanco MO, et al. Second surgery for recurrent glioblastoma: a concise overview of the current literature. Clin Neurol Neurosurg 2016;142:60–4.

27. Stupp R, Mason WP, van den Bent MJ, et al. Radiotherapy plus concomitant and adjuvant temozolomide for glioblastoma. N Engl J Med 2005;352(10):987–96.

28. Stupp R, Newlands E. New approaches for temozolomide therapy: use in newly diagnosed glioma. Semin Oncol 2001;28(4 Suppl 13):19–23.

29. Dubrow R, Darefsky AS, Jacobs DI, et al. Time trends in glioblastoma multiforme survival: the role of temozolomide. Neuro Oncol 2013;15(12):1750–61.

30. Stupp R, Taillibert S, Kanner AA, et al. Maintenance therapy with tumor-treating fields plus temozolomide vs temozolomide alone for glioblastoma: a randomized clinical trial. JAMA 2015;314(23):2535–43.

31. Ortega A, Sarmiento JM, Ly D, et al. Multiple resections and survival of recurrent glioblastoma patients in the temozolomide era. J Clin Neurosci 2016;24:105–11.

32. Stummer W, Pichlmeier U, Meinel T, et al. Fluorescence-guided surgery with 5-aminolevulinic acid

for resection of malignant glioma: a randomised controlled multicentre phase III trial. Lancet Oncol 2006;7(5):392–401.

33. Stummer W, Reulen H-J, Meinel T, et al. Extent of resection and survival in glioblastoma multiforme: identification of and adjustment for bias. Neurosurgery 2008;62(3):564–76 [discussion: 564–76].

34. Lacroix M, Abi-Said D, Fourney DR, et al. A multivariate analysis of 416 patients with glioblastoma multiforme: prognosis, extent of resection, and survival. J Neurosurg 2001;95(2):190–8.

35. Chaichana KL, Jusue-Torres I, Navarro-Ramirez R, et al. Establishing percent resection and residual volume thresholds affecting survival and recurrence for patients with newly diagnosed intracranial glioblastoma. Neuro Oncol 2014;16(1):113–22.

36. Orringer D, Lau D, Khatri S, et al. Extent of resection in patients with glioblastoma: limiting factors, perception of resectability, and effect on survival. J Neurosurg 2012;117(5):851–9.

37. Grabowski MM, Recinos PF, Nowacki AS, et al. Residual tumor volume versus extent of resection: predictors of survival after surgery for glioblastoma. J Neurosurg 2014;121(5):1115–23.

38. McGirt MJ, Chaichana KL, Gathinji M, et al. Independent association of extent of resection with survival in patients with malignant brain astrocytoma. J Neurosurg 2009;110(1):156–62.

39. McGirt MJ, Mukherjee D, Chaichana KL, et al. Association of surgically acquired motor and language deficits on overall survival after resection of glioblastoma multiforme. Neurosurgery 2009;65(3):463–9 [discussion: 469–70].

40. Yong RL, Lonser RR. Surgery for glioblastoma multiforme: striking a balance. World Neurosurg 2011; 76(6):528–30.

41. Gulati S, Jakola AS, Nerland US, et al. The risk of getting worse: surgically acquired deficits, perioperative complications, and functional outcomes after primary resection of glioblastoma. World Neurosurg 2011;76(6):572–9.

42. Stark AM, Nabavi A, Mehdorn HM, et al. Glioblastoma multiforme-report of 267 cases treated at a single institution. Surg Neurol 2005;63(2):162–9 [discussion: 169].

43. Helseth R, Helseth E, Johannesen TB, et al. Overall survival, prognostic factors, and repeated surgery in a consecutive series of 516 patients with glioblastoma multiforme. Acta Neurol Scand 2010;122(3): 159–67.

44. Chaichana KL, Zadnik P, Weingart JD, et al. Multiple resections for patients with glioblastoma: prolonging survival. J Neurosurg 2013;118(4):812–20.

45. Hong B, Wiese B, Bremer M, et al. Multiple microsurgical resections for repeated recurrence of glioblastoma multiforme. Am J Clin Oncol 2013;36(3): 261–8.

46. Park JK, Hodges T, Arko L, et al. Scale to predict survival after surgery for recurrent glioblastoma multiforme. J Clin Oncol 2010;28(24):3838–43.

47. Park C-K, Kim JH, Nam D-H, et al. A practical scoring system to determine whether to proceed with surgical resection in recurrent glioblastoma. Neuro Oncol 2013;15(8):1096–101.

48. Ringel F, Pape H, Sabel M, et al. Clinical benefit from resection of recurrent glioblastomas: results of a multicenter study including 503 patients with recurrent glioblastomas undergoing surgical resection. Neuro Oncol 2016;18(1):96–104.

49. Brandes AA, Bartolotti M, Tosoni A, et al. Patient outcomes following second surgery for recurrent glioblastoma. Future Oncol 2016;12(8):1039–44.

50. Filippini G, Falcone C, Boiardi A, et al. Prognostic factors for survival in 676 consecutive patients with newly diagnosed primary glioblastoma. Neuro Oncol 2008;10(1):79–87.

51. Franceschi E, Bartolotti M, Tosoni A, et al. The effect of re-operation on survival in patients with recurrent glioblastoma. Anticancer Res 2015;35(3):1743–8.

52. Kim HR, Kim KH, Kong D-S, et al. Outcome of salvage treatment for recurrent glioblastoma. J Clin Neurosci 2015;22(3):468–73.

53. Ma X, Lv Y, Liu J, et al. Survival analysis of 205 patients with glioblastoma multiforme: clinical characteristics, treatment and prognosis in China. J Clin Neurosci 2009;16(12):1595–8.

54. Sughrue ME, Sheean T, Bonney PA, et al. Aggressive repeat surgery for focally recurrent primary glioblastoma: outcomes and theoretical framework. Neurosurg Focus 2015;38(3):E17.

55. Tully PA, Gogos AJ, Love C, et al. Reoperation for recurrent glioblastoma and its association with survival benefit. Neurosurgery 2016;79(5):678–89.

56. Bloch O, Han SJ, Cha S, et al. Impact of extent of resection for recurrent glioblastoma on overall survival: clinical article. J Neurosurg 2012;117(6): 1032–8.

57. Quick J, Gessler F, Dutzmann S, et al. Benefit of tumor resection for recurrent glioblastoma. J Neurooncol 2014;117(2):365–72.

58. Oppenlander ME, Wolf AB, Snyder LA, et al. An extent of resection threshold for recurrent glioblastoma and its risk for neurological morbidity. J Neurosurg 2014;120(4):846–53.

59. De Bonis P, Fiorentino A, Anile C, et al. The impact of repeated surgery and adjuvant therapy on survival for patients with recurrent glioblastoma. Clin Neurol Neurosurg 2013;115(7):883–6.

60. Mandl ES, Dirven CMF, Buis DR, et al. Repeated surgery for glioblastoma multiforme: only in combination with other salvage therapy. Surg Neurol 2008; 69(5):506–9 [discussion: 509].

61. Wright RW, Brand RA, Dunn W, et al. How to write a systematic review. Clin Orthop 2007;455:23–9.

62. Archavlis E, Tselis N, Birn G, et al. Combined salvage therapies for recurrent glioblastoma multiforme: Evaluation of an interdisciplinary treatment algorithm. J Neurooncol 2014;119(2):387–95.

63. Bekar A, Ozgur Taskapilioglu M, Morali Güler T, et al. Effect of reoperation on survival of patients with glioblastoma. J Neurol Sci 2012;29(1):110–6.

64. Chen MW, Morsy AA, Liang S, Ng WH. Re-do Craniotomy for Recurrent Grade IV Glioblastomas: Impact and Outcomes from the National Neuroscience Institute Singapore. World Neurosurg 2016;87:439–45.

65. McGirt MJ, Chaichana KL, Gathinji M, et al. Independent association of extent of resection with survival in patients with malignant brain astrocytoma. J Neurosurg 2008;110(1):156–62.

66. McNamara MG, Lwin Z, Jiang H, et al. Factors impacting survival following second surgery in patients with glioblastoma in the temozolomide treatment era, incorporating neutrophil/lymphocyte ratio and time to first progression. J Neurooncol 2014; 117(1):147–52.

67. Michaelsen SR, Christensen IJ, Grunnet K, et al. Clinical variables serve as prognostic factors in a model for survival from glioblastoma multiforme: an observational study of a cohort of consecutive non-selected patients from a single institution. BMC Cancer 2013;13:402.

68. Scorsetti M, Navarria P, Pessina F, et al. Multimodality therapy approaches, local and systemic treatment, compared with chemotherapy alone in recurrent glioblastoma. BMC Cancer 2015;15:486.

69. Suchorska B, Weller M, Tabatabai G, et al. Complete resection of contrast-enhancing tumor volume is associated with improved survival in recurrent glioblastoma-results from the DIRECTOR trial. Neuro-Oncol 2016;18(4):549–56.

70. Woernle CM, Péus D, Hofer S, et al. Efficacy of Surgery and Further Treatment of Progressive Glioblastoma. World Neurosurg 2015;84(2):301–7.

71. Woodworth GF, Garzon-Muvdi T, Ye X, et al. Histopathological correlates with survival in reoperated glioblastomas. J Neurooncol 2013;113(3):485–93.

72. Yong RL, Wu T, Mihatov N, et al. Residual tumor volume and patient survival following reoperation for recurrent glioblastoma. J Neurosurg 2014;121(4): 802–9.

Surgical Treatment of Trigeminal Neuralgia

Sarah K.B. Bick, MD*, Emad N. Eskandar, MD

KEYWORDS

- Trigeminal neuralgia • Microvascular decompression • Percutaneous radiofrequency rhizotomy
- Percutaneous glycerol rhizotomy • Percutaneous balloon compression

KEY POINTS

- Microvascular decompression offers superior long-term pain outcomes for patients with type I trigeminal neuralgia; however, it is associated with the highest rate of serious complications.
- For patients with recurrent pain after microvascular decompression or who are poor operative candidates, percutaneous radiofrequency rhizotomy is the best option among the percutaneous procedures.
- Percutaneous radiofrequency rhizotomy offers the best initial and long-term pain response rates and has the advantage of being able to selectively target affected trigeminal divisions.
- Stereotactic radiosurgery may be useful in patients who fail multiple operative procedures or who have multiple sclerosis–associated trigeminal neuralgia.

INTRODUCTION

Trigeminal neuralgia (TN) is characterized by severe, episodic pain in the distribution of the trigeminal nerve. Type I TN is characterized by episodic lancinating pain, and type II TN has a constant pain component. A variety of methods are used to measure pain severity in TN, with one of the most common being the Barrow Neurologic Institute (BNI) pain scale, which ranges from a score of I indicating no pain and not taking any medications to V indicating severe pain with no relief. Although pharmacologic treatment with medications such as carbamazepine is the first-line therapy, for patients who have resistant pain or who cannot tolerate medications owing to adverse effects a number of operative interventions are available. These include microvascular decompression (MVD), percutaneous radiofrequency rhizotomy (PRR), percutaneous glycerol rhizotomy (PGR), percutaneous balloon compression (PBC), and stereotactic radiosurgery (SRS), including gamma knife radiosurgery (GKRS) or cyberknife.

These procedures have varying success rates and risk profiles. We review the evidence supporting the risks and benefits of the various operative modalities.

MICROVASCULAR DECOMPRESSION
Success Rates

MVD involves performing a suboccipital craniotomy to find and resolve the underlying trigeminal nerve compression (**Fig. 1**). MVD offers excellent pain control results. The rate of initial pain control is 80.3% to 96%.[1–4] One prospective study found that 92.5% of patients were pain free without medication at average 28 month follow-up.[5] In another study at mean of 38 months of follow-up, 85% of patients maintained adequate pain control.[4] At 5 years, 72% to 85% have good pain control.[1–3,6] One of the largest studies of MVD with long-term follow-up found that at 10 years 70% of patients had complete pain relief and 4% had partial pain relief.[7] Another study with very long-term follow-up found that at 15 years 73.4%

Disclosure Statement: The authors have nothing to disclose.
Department of Neurosurgery, Massachusetts General Hospital, Their 4, 55 Fruit Street, Boston, MA 02114, USA
* Corresponding author.
E-mail address: sbick@partners.org

neurosurgery.theclinics.com

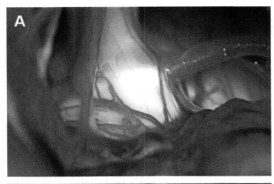
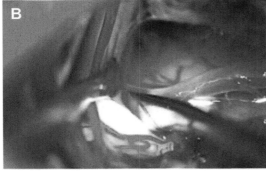
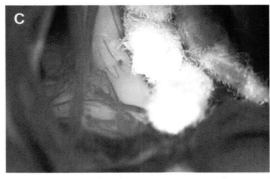

Fig. 1. Microvascular decompression. A suboccipital craniotomy is performed to expose the borders of the transverse and sigmoid sinuses. The dura is incised and cerebrospinal fluid carefully drained to expose the cerebellopontine angle. (*A*) The trigeminal nerve is seen draped over a compressive artery. (*B*) The artery is dissected away from the nerve. (*C*) Teflon pledgets are placed between the nerve and compressive artery to maintain their separation.

of patients were pain free.[8] Pain relief after MVD is generally instantaneous, although a delay of up to 1 month before the benefit is evident has been reported.[4,9]

MVD has highest success rates in patients with type I TN.[9] Type II TN may have more advanced underlying nerve damage contributing to worse immediate and long-term outcomes.[2,9,10] Arterial versus venous compression may also be associated with TN type and is associated with better

outcomes after MVD.[10,11] In patients with episodic pain that evolves into constant pain, MVD may still provide significant pain relief, especially for the episodic component of pain.[12] However, freedom from pain is less likely if constant pain comprises more than 50% of the pain experienced.[12]

A greater degree of neurovascular compression has been associated with better long-term outcomes in some studies,[8] as has the presence of preoperative trigger points.[2] Patients with immediate postoperative pain relief, male gender, absence of venous compression, and shorter disease duration may have better outcomes.[7,13] Bilateral pain is correlated with worse outcomes.[2] MVD is less effective for multiple sclerosis (MS)-related TN, with 50% experiencing complete pain relief and 10% partial pain relief at a mean of 2 years of follow-up.[4]

Because MVD is more invasive than other surgical procedures for TN, its safety and efficacy in older patients has been debated. One study suggested that although all ages had the same rate of initial pain relief (>95%), patients over age 60 had a shorter time to recurrence.[14] However, the older patient group had a longer duration of symptoms before surgery, which may have contributed to worse outcomes. Another study found lower recurrence rates in elderly patients.[15] Older patients may have better outcomes after repeat MVD.[16] Young patients may have worse outcomes after MVD, perhaps related to a lower incidence of arterial compression at the time of surgery.[3,17]

MVD can be successful as a repeat procedure for appropriately selected candidates who have recurrence of TN after initial MVD or other surgical procedure, although rates of pain relief are likely lower than with initial MVD,[3,18] with 90.3% to 93.3% initial complete pain relief,[18,19] 67% success rate at 12 months,[16] and 42% excellent results at 10 years.[7] Another study that included partial sensory rhizotomy in repeat MVD found 10% good outcome at the 4-year follow-up.[13] Patients with previous ablative procedures have worse outcomes after MVD, with 64% reported excellent outcome at a mean of 5.1 years of follow-up.[13]

Complications

Although MVD is the most invasive operative procedure for TN, in experienced hands the complication rate is relatively low. There is a 4% rate of serious complications.[9] Mortality rate is reported at 0.15% to 0.8%.[7,9,14,20,21] There is a lower complication rate and lower rate of mortality or discharge to other than home with greater hospital and surgeon volume.[21]

MVD has a 1.6% to 22% rate of postoperative trigeminal nerve deficit, with approximately one-half of cases being transient.[4–7,11,14] Facial weakness occurs in 0.6% to 10.6%, with some deficits improving with time.[4–7,11,13,21,22] There is a 1.2% to 6.8% rate of hearing loss.[4,6,7,11,13,23] Monitoring brainstem evoked responses during the procedure may help to decrease this complication, which is often associated with retraction.[23] Two percent experience aseptic meningitis.[6] Hydrocephalus occurs in 0.15%.[7] The reported rate of cerebrospinal fluid (CSF) leak is 1.5% to 4%.[5,7,11,23] Cerebellar infarct or hematoma may occur in 0.075% to 0.68%.[4,7,23] Anesthesia dolorosa is reported at rates from 0% in one large series[7] to 4% in patients who underwent internal neurolysis during MVD.[3]

Two studies using the Nationwide Inpatient Sample found a relationship between mortality and discharge to other than home and age.[21,24] Age also correlates with incidence of cardiac, pulmonary, thromboembolic, and cerebrovascular complications but not with CNS infection, wound complications, cranial nerve deficits, or CSF leak.[15,24] Other studies including a meta analysis of studies examining MVD and age[25] have reported no difference in complication rates.[6,26–28]

Patients with prior MVD may have a higher complication rate.[6] Trigeminal nerve complications may be higher and have been reported at 8.3% to 32% after repeat MVD.[7,13,16,18] Hearing loss occurs in 6.7%.[19]

PERCUTANEOUS TREATMENTS
Percutaneous Radiofrequency Rhizotomy

Success rates
Percutaneous procedures use a needle to access the gasserian ganglion and introduce injury via heat, chemical injury, or mechanical compression (**Fig. 2**). Reported outcomes after percutaneous procedures are more variable, depending in part on the outcome measure used. Initial response rate to PRR is reported at 97.6% to 99%.[29,30] At 6 months, there is a 83.3% to 89.9% response rate.[29,31] Reports of recurrence rates vary from 38.2% at 1 year[32] to 10% at 6.5 years follow-up.[30] A large series reported 41% of patients retaining complete pain control after 20 years.[29]

Type I TN is associated with better outcomes after PRR,[9,31] although bilateral pain and comorbid psychiatric conditions may be associated with worse outcomes.[31] An advantage of PRR is that it may allow more selective targeting of trigeminal nerve distributions than other percutaneous procedures.[31] PRR is effective for MS-related TN, but requires the production of anesthesia in the affected trigeminal divisions.[30]

Complications
Hypesthesia lasting at least 1 month occurs in 3.3%.[31] There is a 5.7% to 17.3% rate of decreased corneal sensation with an 0.6% to 1.9% rate of keratitis.[29,30,32] Four percent of patients experience masseter weakness.[29] There is a 0.6% to 0.8% rate of anesthesia dolorosa.[29,32] PRR damages small unmyelinated pain fibers contributing to adverse effects.[33] Higher temperatures may be associated with the rate of hypesthesia.[20]

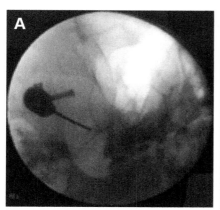
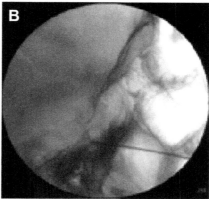

Fig. 2. Percutaneous procedures. Percutaneous radiofrequency rhizotomy (PRR), percutaneous glycerol rhizotomy (PGR), and percutaneous balloon compression (PBC) all involve entry of a needle through the foramen ovale to introduce injury to the trigeminal nerve. A needle is introduced 2.5 cm lateral to the labial fissure. (*A*) The needle is advanced medial to the ramus of the jaw into the foramen ovale using oblique view fluoroscopic imaging. (*B*) A lateral radiograph is used to confirm the location of the needle. Once positioned, trigeminal nerve injury is performed via radiofrequency ablation (PRR), glycerol injection (PGR), or mechanical compression (PBC).

Percutaneous Glycerol Rhizotomy

Success rates

Seventy-one percent to 97.9% of patients have immediate and complete pain relief.[9,30,34,35] PGR has mean duration 11 months.[9] At 1 year to 13.5 months of follow-up, there is a 53% to 63% rate of pain control.[32,36,37] At 54 months, the recurrence rate is 72%.[38] At 5 years, 56.5% recur.[30] Another study reported a 10-year recurrence rate at 18.8%, with most recurrences occurring within the first 3 years.[34]

High preoperative pain score, postoperative hypoesthesia,[34,37,39,40] and presence of pain-free intervals are correlated with outcome after PGR.[9] CSF outflow during the procedure is correlated with lower recurrence rates.[34] Three or more prior PGRs are correlated with shorter time to recurrence.[39]

There are reports of similar[9] and worse outcomes for type II TN after PGR, with 100% experiencing recurrence within 1 year.[37] PGR may relieve the episodic but not constant pain component in type II TN.[37]

MS-related TN may have a higher recurrence rate, with 78% recurring within a mean of 13 months.[37] Another study found 78% initial complete pain relief with 59% recurrence at a mean of 17 months.[41] Outcomes were better in patients with hypesthesia.[41]

Complications

Aseptic meningitis occurs in 0.12% to 3% of patients[34,35,37,39] and bacterial meningitis in 1.5% to 1.7%.[37,39] Carotid puncture occurs in 0.77%.[39] Penetration of buccal mucosa occurs at a rate of 1.5%,[39] and cheek hematoma in 7%.[39] Hypesthesia occurs in 23.3% to 72%,[30,34,37–39] with higher rates in patients undergoing repeat procedures.[38] Decreased corneal sensation occurs in 6.3% to 15%.[32,34,37] There is a 1.9% rate of hearing loss.[39]

Percutaneous Balloon Compression

Success

There is a 82% to 93.8% initial response rate.[30,35,42] At 1 year, there is a 25.4% recurrence rate.[32] At a mean of 4 years, long-term pain control is 69.4%.[43] Another study found a 20% recurrence rate at 5 years. At a mean of 10.7 years of follow-up, there is a 31.9% recurrence rate.[44] Time to symptom recurrence may be related to balloon compression time and to duration and extent of hypesthesia.[40,45]

Repeat PBC for recurrent TN may be effective with 83% to 93.8% of patients having immediate pain relief.[45,46] At a median of 64.8 months of follow-up, 54.5% remained free of pain.[46]

Complications

PBC has a high rate of hypesthesia, with 89% to 100% of patients having initial numbness[14,44] and 4.6% to 40% having some persistent symptoms.[30,42,44,47] Trigeminal nerve dysfunction may be proportional to the rate and duration of balloon compression.[30,43,47] There is a 0% to 3.1% rate of decreased corneal sensation.[43,44,48] PBC selectively injures medium and large myelinated pain fibers, preserving small myelinated and unmyelinated fibers, which help to preserve corneal sensation.[33]

Hearing loss occurs in 2.4% to 6.3%,[48] whereas 1.2% to 12% experience masseter weakness.[30,35,42–44] Cheek hematoma occurs in 3.5% to 6.7%.[42,43] Aseptic meningitis is reported in 0.7% and bacterial meningitis in 0.7% to 1%.[42,48] Pseudoaneurysm may occur in 1%.[48] PBC may have a higher rate of trigeminal reflex bradycardia and hypotension than other percutaneous procedures,[33] potentially making it less suitable for patients with underlying cardiac comorbidities.

Patients undergoing repeat PBC may have a higher rate of jaw weakness and decreased corneal sensation.[45,46] There is a high rate of trigeminal nerve dysfunction, with 55% experiencing persistent numbness.[46] One study of PBC after previous other failed procedure found a 7% rate of ipsilateral facial weakness and 0% to 3.4% of anesthesia dolorosa.[44,46]

Stereotactic Radiosurgery

Success rates

After GKRS 79% to 91.8% of patients have initial pain improvement.[49–53] Pain improvement after GKRS is delayed, with 10 days to 3.4 months weeks until pain relief.[49–57] Duration of symptoms is associated with latency of response.[52] Earlier response may be associated with durability of response.[57] Median duration of pain relief is reported at 32 months to 4.1 years.[49,58] At 1 year, 75% to 90% have BNI I to IIIB pain scores.[57] At 3 years, 70% maintain improvement in pain, with 34% pain free without medication.[53,56] At 5 to 5.6 years, 44% to 65% of patients retain pain relief.[49,57] Another study reported 76% are pain free at 7 years.[54] At 10 years, 30% to 51.5% maintain good pain relief.[51,59] In a large cohort of TN patients who underwent GKRS, 29% ultimately required further procedures for pain control.[51]

Patients who have not previously undergone surgery have more durable pain relief.[49,50,54] Initial medication responsiveness is also a positive predictor of outcome.[54] Some studies report no difference in response rates between different radiation doses.[49] With a constant radiation dose, the dose rate may be associated with pain relief outcomes after GKRS.[58] Older age may also be associated with better outcomes,[51,53,56,58] as is shorter duration of symptoms.[52] Postprocedure facial numbness is associated with pain outcomes.[50,51,54,57,60] Although neurovascular compression does not predict response to GKRS, dose to site of compression and distance from isocenter to site of compression are associated with pain relief.[61] Type I TN patients are more likely to have initial response and less likely to relapse after GKRS.[51,53,57] In bilateral TN GKRS has 80% pain control rate at 12 months and 65% at 36 months.[62]

Repeat GKRS may be effective in patients who have recurrence after initial GKRS, with 60% to 100% with initial pain response after repeat procedure,[63,64] with 75% maintaining pain freedom at 1 year[64] and a median duration of response of 3.8 years.[60] Patients who have a good response to initial GKS have better response to repeat procedure, as do those with hypesthesia after initial procedure.[60] Radiation dose may be correlated with response to repeat GKRS.[64] In patients undergoing a third GKRS procedure, 47.1% had initial BNI I scores and 47.1% BI II to IIIb scores at a mean of 2.9 months after the procedure, with 35.3% maintaining BNI I and 41.2% BNI II to IIIb scores at a mean of 22.9 months of follow-up.[65]

Patients who underwent GKRS after failing previous surgical treatment for TN had 81% BNI I to IIIb rates of pain control at 1 year.[66] In another study, patients undergoing GKRS for recurrent pain after initial MVD, GKRS, or PRR found 66% with a BNI score of I to IIIb at a median of 3 years of follow-up.[67] At 6 years, there is a 58% rate of BNI I to IIIb pain control.[66] Hypesthesia is associated with better outcomes,[66,67] as is fewer previous interventions.[66] In patients who had previously undergone MVD, 77.8% achieved initial pain freedom after median 14 days, significantly faster than in the general TN population.[68] At 10 years, 44.3% remained pain free without medication.[68]

After cyberknife radiosurgery, 61.9% to 87.2% of patients have initial pain relief.[69,70] There is a 19-month median time to pain recurrence.[69] At a median of 24 to 28 months of follow-up, 72% of patients have good pain outcomes.[69,70] At 2 years of follow-up, 72% of patients had good pain outcomes.[70] Hypesthesia is associated with better outcome.[69] A higher initial pain score may be associated with better pain outcomes.[70]

Complications

There is a 6% to 42% rate of hypesthesia after GKRS, with similar rates after cyberknife radiosurgery.[49–52,54,56,58,69] Hypesthesia may be delayed, occurring at a median of 12 months.[50] Hypesthesia is dose dependent and may be related to the

proximity of the target to the brainstem.[53,57] Anesthesia dolorosa has been reported in 0.2%.[51]

After repeat GKRS, there is a higher rate of hypesthesia at 11% to 80%[53,64] and a 6.6% rate of corneal dryness.[60] A cumulative radiation dose of more than 115 Gy may be related to hypesthesia.[64] A reported 1.3% of patients experienced anesthesia dolorosa.[60]

When GKRS is performed after initial failed MVD, GKRS, or PRR, there is a 9.3% to 26% rate of new facial numbness,[66] which is associated with radiation dose.[67] Anesthesia dolorosa occurs in 0.5%.[66]

SUMMARY

Available treatment options for TN have different risks and benefits stemming from their differing success rates and complication profiles (**Table 1**). A careful consideration of these factors will help to determine which procedure is more most appropriate for a specific situation.

MVD offers high initial response rates as well as the longest durability. Studies directly comparing MVD with other treatment modalities have found the most favorable pain outcomes after MVD. PRR and MVD have similar initial response rates, but there is a significantly longer response after MVD.[20,71] PRR patients are more likely to require a subsequent procedure for TN-related pain than those undergoing MVD or SRS.[72] A study of a national discharge registry from the Netherlands comparing MVD, open partial sensory rhizotomy, and PRR found that MVD had the lowest 1-year readmission rate[73]; however, PRR had the lowest complication rate.[73] PRR does have a higher rate of hypesthesia than SRS or MVD.[72,74]

Several studies have reported that cost effectiveness is best for PRR, followed by MVD, followed by SRS.[72,75] However, this calculation does not take into account the cost of multiple additional procedures that may be required in young patients with TN given the higher recurrence rate after percutaneous procedures, considering the relatively short follow-up of the studies. Another study found that patients undergoing MVD followed by SRS followed by PRR required the fewest number of procedures to achieve pain relief.[74]

In a group of patients who underwent GKRS or MVD based on their own preference, a significantly greater percentage of those who underwent MVD had initial BNI scores of I to III, and additionally MVD provided more immediate pain relief.[76] Recurrence rates were similar between the 2 groups.[76] A study in patients over 65 years of age found similar results.[77] Other studies have

Table 1
Success rates and complication profiles for TN treatment options

Procedure	Initial Response Rate (%)	Long-Term Response Rates (%)	Predictors of Response	Complications (%)
Microvascular decompression	80.3–96	1 y: 84 5 y: 72–85 10 y: 74	+ Type I TN, arterial neurovascular compression, preoperative trigger points, shorter disease duration - Bilateral TN, MS associated TN, type II TN	CN V: 1.6–22 CN VII: 0.6–10.6 CN VIII: 1.2–6.8 Anesthesia dolorosa: 0–4 CSF leak: 1.5–4 Cerebellar infarct/hematoma: 0.075–0.68 Mortality: 0.15–0.8
Percutaneous radiofrequency rhizotomy	97.6–99	1 y: 61.8 5 y: 57.7 10 y: 52.3 20 y: 41	+ type I TN - Bilateral symptoms	CN V: 3.3 Decreased corneal sensation: 5.7–17.3 Keratitis 0.6–1.9 Anesthesia dolorosa: 0.6–0.8
PGR	71–97.9	1 y: 53–63 5 y: 43.5	+ High preoperative pain score, postoperative hypoesthesia, presence of pain-free intervals - ≥3 previous PGRs	CN V: 23.3–72 Decreased corneal sensation 6.3–15 CN VIII: 1.9 Aseptic meningitis 0.12–3 Bacterial meningitis 1.5–1.7
Percutaneous balloon compression	82–93.8	1 y: 74.6 5 y: 69–80 10 y: 68.1		CN V: 4.6–40 Decreased corneal sensation: 0–3.1 CN VIII: 2.4–6.3 Aseptic meningitis: 0.7 Bacterial meningitis: 0.7–1
Stereotactic radiosurgery	79–91.8 (delayed 10 d–3.4 mo)	1 y: 75–90 5 y: 44–65 10 y: 30–51.5	+ Earlier response, no previous TN surgery, medication responsiveness, postprocedure facial numbness	CN V: 6–42 Anesthesia dolorosa: 0.2

Abbreviations: +, positively correlated with response; −, negatively correlated with response; CN, cranial nerve; CSF, cerebrospinal fluid; MS, multiple sclerosis; PGR, percutaneous glycerol rhizotomy; TN, trigeminal neuralgia.

reported longer durability of pain relief after MVD compared with GKRS.[78,79] Patients treated with GKRS have a higher incidence of facial numbness and corneal anesthesia,[79] whereas patients who underwent MVD had higher rates of facial weakness and hearing loss.[76]

A systematic treatment algorithm whereby MVD was performed in patients younger than 70 years of age and PRR was performed in older patients or for those in whom MVD had previously failed had good long-term outcomes, with 93% experiencing significant pain relief within 1 month of the procedure, with 78% retaining significant relief at an average of 1.2 years of follow-up.[71]

Although MVD has higher rates of serious complications, including facial weakness, hearing loss, cerebellar infarct or hematoma, and CSF leak, as well as higher mortality than other procedures, in experienced hands the incidence of these complications remains relatively low. Given the superior long-term response rate of MVD, it remains the initial treatment of choice in patients with type I TN, including older patients who are acceptable operative candidates.

Percutaneous procedures offer an alternative treatment in patients in whom MVD has failed or in whom systemic comorbidities make the operative risk of MVD unacceptably high. Among the percutaneous procedures, PRR offers excellent initial and long-term response rates and the advantage of the ability to selectively target affected trigeminal divisions. A systematic review examining ablative therapies for TN found that PRR had the highest rates of long-term complete pain relief.[80] Direct comparison has suggested that PRR may have a longer duration of efficacy than PGR.[9,33] However, hypesthesia may be more common after PRR than PGR.[9] PGR and PBC have similar initial success rates and durations of effect.[35,40] PBC has a higher complication rate than PGR or PRR, and has a high rate of hypesthesia.[32,40]

SRS may play a role for TN patients who are poor operative candidates or who have pain that has been resistant to other operative modalities. SRS has a lower complication rate than the percutaneous procedures and also has lower rates of hypesthesia and anesthesia dolorosa.[80] One downside of this treatment modality is the latency of the response. SRS may also play a role in MS-related TN. Of the percutaneous procedures, PRR has the best effect for MS related TN[30]; however, SRS may be the most effective treatment modality for this patient group.[33]

REFERENCES

1. Pamir M, Peker S. Microvascular decompression for trigeminal neuralgia: a long-term follow-up study. Minim Invasive Neurosurg 2006;49(6):342–6.
2. Tyler-Kabara EC, Kassam AB, Horowitz MH, et al. Predictors of outcome in surgically managed patients with typical and atypical trigeminal neuralgia: comparison of results following microvascular decompression. J Neurosurg 2002;96(3):527–31.
3. Ko AL, Ozpinar A, Lee A, et al. Long-term efficacy and safety of internal neurolysis for trigeminal neuralgia without neurovascular compression. J Neurosurg 2015;122(5):1048–57.
4. Broggi G, Ferroli P, Franzini A, et al. Microvascular decompression for trigeminal neuralgia: comments on a series of 250 cases, including 10 patients with multiple sclerosis. J Neurol Neurosurg Psychiatr 2000;68(1):59–64.
5. Chakravarthi PS, Ghanta R, Kattimani V. Microvascular decompression treatment for trigeminal neuralgia. J Craniofac Surg 2011;22(3):894–8.
6. Pollock BE, Stein KJ. Posterior fossa exploration for trigeminal neuralgia patients older than 70 years of age. Neurosurgery 2011;69(6):1255–9.
7. Barker FG, Jannetta PJ, Bissonette DJ, et al. The long-term outcome of microvascular decompression for trigeminal neuralgia. N Engl J Med 1996;334(17):1077–83.
8. Sindou M, Leston J, Decullier E, et al. Microvascular decompression for primary trigeminal neuralgia: long-term effectiveness and prognostic factors in a series of 362 consecutive patients with clear-cut neurovascular conflicts who underwent pure decompression. J Neurosurg 2007;107(6):1144–53.
9. Degn J, Brennum J. Surgical treatment of trigeminal neuralgia. Results from the use of glycerol injection, microvascular decompression, and rhizotomia. Acta Neurochir 2010;152(12):2125–32.
10. Miller JP, Magill ST, Acar F, et al. Predictors of long-term success after microvascular decompression for trigeminal neuralgia. J Neurosurg 2009;110(4):620–6.
11. Günther T, Gerganov VM, Stieglitz L, et al. Microvascular decompression for trigeminal neuralgia in the elderly. Neurosurgery 2009;65(3):477–82.
12. Sandell T, Eide PK. Effect of microvascular decompression in trigeminal neuralgia patients with or without constant pain. Neurosurgery 2008;63(1):93–9 [discussion: 99–100].
13. Bederson JB, Wilson CB. Evaluation of microvascular decompression and partial sensory rhizotomy in 252 cases of trigeminal neuralgia. J Neurosurg 1989;71(3):359–67.
14. Ashkan K, Marsh H. Microvascular decompression for trigeminal neuralgia in the elderly: a review of the safety and efficacy. Neurosurgery 2004;55(4):840–50.
15. Phan K, Rao PJ, Dexter M. Microvascular decompression for elderly patients with trigeminal neuralgia. J Clin Neurosci 2016;29(C):7–14.
16. Bakker NA, Van Dijk JMC, Immenga S, et al. Repeat microvascular decompression for recurrent idiopathic trigeminal neuralgia. J Neurosurg 2014;121(4):936–9.
17. Bahgat D, Ray DK, Raslan AM, et al. Trigeminal neuralgia in young adults. J Neurosurg 2011;1–6. http://dx.doi.org/10.3171/2010.10.JNS10781.
18. Theodros D, Rory Goodwin C, Bender MT, et al. Efficacy of primary microvascular decompression versus subsequent microvascular decompression for trigeminal neuralgia. J Neurosurg 2016;1–7. http://dx.doi.org/10.3171/2016.5.JNS151692.
19. Yang D-B, Jiang D-Y, Chen H-C, et al. Second microvascular decompression for trigeminal neuralgia in recurrent cases after microvascular decompression. J Craniofac Surg 2015;26(2):491–4.
20. Tronnier VM, Rasche D, Hamer J, et al. Treatment of idiopathic trigeminal neuralgia: comparison of long-term outcome after radiofrequency rhizotomy and microvascular decompression. Neurosurgery 2001;48(6):1261–7 [discussion: 1267–8].

21. Kalkanis SN, Eskandar EN, Carter BS, et al. Micro-vascular decompression surgery in the united states, 1996 to 2000: mortality rates, morbidity rates, and the effects of hospital and surgeon volumes. Neurosurgery 2003;52(6):1251–62.

22. Chang JW, Chang JH, Park YG, et al. Microvascular decompression in trigeminal neuralgia: a correlation of three-dimensional time-of-flight magnetic reso-nance angiography and surgical findings. Stereo-tact Funct Neurosurg 2000;74(3–4):167–74.

23. McLaughlin MR, Jannetta PJ, Clyde BL, et al. Micro-vascular decompression of cranial nerves: lessons learned after 4400 operations. J Neurosurg 1999; 90(1):1–8.

24. Rughani AI, Dumont TM, Lin C-T, et al. Safety of microvascular decompression for trigeminal neural-gia in the elderly. Clinical article. J Neurosurg 2011;115(2):202–9.

25. Sekula RF, Frederickson AM, Jannetta PJ, et al. Microvascular decompression for elderly patients with trigeminal neuralgia: a prospective study and systematic review with meta-analysis. J Neurosurg 2011;114(1):172–9.

26. Javadpour M, Eldridge PR, Varma TRK, et al. Micro-vascular decompression for trigeminal neuralgia in patients over 70 years of age. Neurology 2003; 60(3):520.

27. Sekula RF Jr, Marchan EM, Fletcher LH, et al. Microvascular decompression for trigeminal neu-ralgia in elderly patients. J Neurosurg 2008; 108(4):689–91.

28. Zhao H, Tang Y, Zhang X, et al. Microvascular decompression for idiopathic primary trigeminal neuralgia in patients over 75 years of age. J Craniofac Surg 2016;27(5):1295–7.

29. Kanpolat Y, Savas A, Bekar A, et al. Percutaneous controlled radiofrequency trigeminal rhizotomy for the treatment of idiopathic trigeminal neuralgia: 25-year experience with 1,600 patients. Neurosurgery 2001;48(3):524–32 [discussion: 532–4].

30. Fraioli B, Esposito V, Guidetti B, et al. Treatment of trigeminal neuralgia by thermocoagulation, glyc-erolization, and percutaneous compression of the gasserian ganglion and/or retrogasserian rootlets: long-term results and therapeutic protocol. Neuro-surgery 1989;24(2):239–45.

31. Jin HS, Shin JY, Kim Y-C, et al. Predictive factors associated with success and failure for radiofre-quency thermocoagulation in patients with trigemi-nal neuralgia. Pain Physician 2015;18(6):537–45.

32. Noorani I, Lodge A, Vajramani G, et al. Comparing percutaneous treatments of trigeminal neuralgia: 19 years of experience in a single centre. Stereotact Funct Neurosurg 2016;94(2):75–85.

33. Cheng JS, Lim DA, Chang EF, et al. A review of percutaneous treatments for trigeminal neuralgia. Oper Neurosurg 2014;10(1):25–33.

34. Chen L, Xu M, Zou Y. Treatment of trigeminal neuralgia with percutaneous glycerol injection into Meckel's cavity: experience in 4012 patients. Cell Biochem Biophys 2010;58(2):85–9.

35. Asplund P, Blomstedt P, Bergenheim AT. Percu-taneous balloon compression vs percutaneous retrogasserian glycerol rhizotomy for the primary treatment of trigeminal neuralgia. Neurosurgery 2016;78(3):421–8.

36. Bergenheim AT, Hariz MI, Laitinen LV, et al. Relation between sensory disturbance and outcome after ret-rogasserian glycerol rhizotomy. Acta Neurochir 1991;111(3–4):114–8.

37. Burchiel KJ. Percutaneous retrogasserian glycerol rhizolysis in the management of trigeminal neuralgia. J Neurosurg 1988;69(3):361–6.

38. Fujimaki T, Fukushima T, Miyazaki S. Percutaneous retrogasserian glycerol injection in the management of trigeminal neuralgia: long-term follow-up results. J Neurosurg 1990;73(2):212–6.

39. Blomstedt PC, Bergenheim AT. Technical difficulties and perioperative complications of retrogasserian glycerol rhizotomy for trigeminal neuralgia. Stereo-tact Funct Neurosurg 2003;79(3–4):168–81.

40. Kouzounias K, Lind G, Schechtmann G, et al. Com-parison of percutaneous balloon compression and glycerol rhizotomy for the treatment of trigeminal neuralgia. J Neurosurg 2010;113(3):486–92.

41. Pickett GE, Bisnaire D, Ferguson GG. Percutaneous retrogasserian glycerol rhizotomy in the treatment of tic douloureux associated with multiple sclerosis. Neurosurgery 2005;56(3):537–45.

42. Lobato RD, Rivas JJ, Sarabia R, et al. Percutaneous microcompression of the gasserian ganglion for tri-geminal neuralgia. J Neurosurg 1990;72(4):546–53.

43. Abdennebi B, Bouatta F, Chitti M, et al. Percuta-neous balloon compression of the Gasserian gan-glion in trigeminal neuralgia. Long-term results in 150 cases. Acta Neurochir 1995;136(1–2):72–4.

44. Skirving DJ, Dan NG. A 20-year review of percuta-neous balloon compression of the trigeminal gan-glion. J Neurosurg 2001;94(6):913–7.

45. Chen JF, Tu PH, Lee ST. Repeated percutaneous balloon compression for recurrent trigeminal neural-gia: a long-term study. World Neurosurg 2012;77(2): 352–6.

46. Omeis I, Smith D, Kim S, et al. Percutaneous balloon compression for the treatment of recurrent trigeminal neuralgia: long-term outcome in 29 patients. Stereo-tact Funct Neurosurg 2008;86(4):259–65.

47. Lichtor T, Mullan JF. A 10-year follow-up review of percutaneous microcompression of the trigeminal ganglion. J Neurosurg 1990;72(1):49–54.

48. de Siqueira SRDT, da Nóbrega JCM, de Siqueira JTT, et al. Frequency of postoperative com-plications after balloon compression for idiopathic trigeminal neuralgia: prospective study. Oral Surg

Oral Med Oral Pathol Oral Radiol Endod 2006; 102(5):e39–45.

49. Dhople AA, Adams JR, Maggio WW, et al. Long-term outcomes of Gamma Knife radiosurgery for classic trigeminal neuralgia: implications of treatment and critical review of the literature. Clinical article. J Neurosurg 2009;111(2):351–8.

50. Régis J, Tuleasca C, Resseguier N, et al. Long-term safety and efficacy of Gamma Knife surgery in classical trigeminal neuralgia: a 497-patient historical cohort study. J Neurosurg 2016;124(4):1079–87.

51. Kondziolka D, Zorro O, Lobato-Polo J, et al. Gamma Knife stereotactic radiosurgery for idiopathic trigeminal neuralgia. J Neurosurg 2010;112(4):758–65.

52. Mousavi SH, Niranjan A, Huang MJ, et al. Early radiosurgery provides superior pain relief for trigeminal neuralgia patients. Neurology 2015;85(24): 2159–65.

53. Taich ZJ, Goetsch SJ, Monaco E, et al. Stereotactic radiosurgery treatment of trigeminal neuralgia: clinical outcomes and prognostic factors. World Neurosurg 2016;90:604–12.e11.

54. Martínez Moreno NE, Gutiérrez-Sárraga J, Rey-Portolés G, et al. Long-term outcomes in the treatment of classical trigeminal neuralgia by gamma knife radiosurgery. Neurosurgery 2016;1–9. http://dx.doi.org/10.1227/NEU.0000000000001404.

55. Park S-H, Hwang S-K. Outcomes of gamma knife radiosurgery for trigeminal neuralgia after a minimum 3-year follow-up. J Clin Neurosci 2011;18(5):645–8.

56. Sheehan J, Pan H-C, Stroila M, et al. Gamma knife surgery for trigeminal neuralgia: outcomes and prognostic factors. J Neurosurg 2005;102(3): 434–41.

57. Wolf A, Kondziolka D. Gamma knife surgery in trigeminal neuralgia. Neurosurg Clin N Am 2016; 27(3):297–304.

58. Lee JYK, Sandhu S, Miller D, et al. Higher dose rate Gamma Knife radiosurgery may provide earlier and longer-lasting pain relief for patients with trigeminal neuralgia. J Neurosurg 2015;123(4):961–8.

59. Régis J, Tuleasca C, Resseguier N, et al. The very long-term outcome of radiosurgery for classical trigeminal neuralgia. Stereotact Funct Neurosurg 2016;94(1):24–32.

60. Helis CA, Lucas JT Jr, Bourland JD, et al. Repeat radiosurgery for trigeminal neuralgia. Neurosurgery 2015;77(5):755–61.

61. Sheehan JP, Ray DK, Monteith S, et al. Gamma Knife radiosurgery for trigeminal neuralgia: the impact of magnetic resonance imaging–detected vascular impingement of the affected nerve. J Neurosurg 2010;113(1):53–8.

62. Raval A, Salluzzo J, Price L, et al. Salvage Gamma Knife Radiosurgery after failed management of bilateral trigeminal neuralgia. Surg Neurol Int 2014;5(1):160.

63. Park S-C, Do Kwon H, Do Lee H, et al. Repeat gamma-knife radiosurgery for refractory or recurrent trigeminal neuralgia with consideration about the optimal second dose. World Neurosurg 2016; 86(C):371–83.

64. Tuleasca C, Carron R, Resseguier N, et al. Repeat Gamma Knife surgery for recurrent trigeminal neuralgia: long-term outcomes and systematic review. J Neurosurg 2014;121(Suppl):210–21.

65. Tempel ZJ, Chivukula S, Monaco EA III, et al. The results of a third Gamma Knife procedure for recurrent trigeminal neuralgia. J Neurosurg 2015;122(1): 169–79.

66. Kano H, Kondziolka D, Yang H-C, et al. Outcome predictors after gamma knife radiosurgery for recurrent trigeminal neuralgia. Neurosurgery 2010;67(6): 1637–45.

67. Huang C-F, Chiou S-Y, Wu M-F, et al. Gamma Knife surgery for recurrent or residual trigeminal neuralgia after a failed initial procedure. J Neurosurg 2010; 113(Suppl):172–7.

68. Tuleasca C, Carron R, Resseguier N, et al. Decreased probability of initial pain cessation in classic trigeminal neuralgia treated with gamma knife surgery in case of previous microvascular decompression. Neurosurgery 2015;77(1):87–95.

69. Karam SD, Tai A, Snider JW, et al. Refractory trigeminal neuralgia treatment outcomes following CyberKnife radiosurgery. Radiat Oncol 2014; 9(1):257.

70. Singh R, Davis J, Sharma S. Stereotactic radiosurgery for trigeminal neuralgia: a retrospective multi-institutional examination of treatment outcomes. Cureus 2016;1–14. http://dx.doi.org/10.7759/cureus.554.

71. Amirnovin R, Neimat JS, Roberts JA, et al. Multimodality treatment of trigeminal neuralgia. Stereotact Funct Neurosurg 2005;83(5–6):197–201.

72. Holland M, Noeller J, Buatti J, et al. The cost-effectiveness of surgery for trigeminal neuralgia in surgically naïve patients: a retrospective study. Clin Neurol Neurosurg 2015;137:34–7.

73. Koopman JSHA, de Vries LM, Dieleman JP, et al. A nationwide study of three invasive treatments for trigeminal neuralgia. Pain 2011;152(3):507–13.

74. Hitchon PW, Holland M, Noeller J, et al. Options in treating trigeminal neuralgia: Experience with 195 patients. Clin Neurol Neurosurg 2016;149:166–70.

75. Sivakanthan S, Van Gompel JJ, Alikhani P, et al. Surgical management of trigeminal neuralgia. Neurosurgery 2014;75(3):220–6.

76. Dai Z-F, Huang Q, Liu H, et al. Efficacy of stereotactic gamma knife surgery and microvascular decompression in the treatment of primary trigeminal neuralgia: a retrospective study of 220 cases from a single center. J Peace Res 2016; 9:535–42.

77. Oh IH, Choi SK, Park BJ, et al. The treatment outcome of elderly patients with idiopathic trigeminal neuralgia : micro-vascular decompression versus gamma knife radiosurgery. J Korean Neurosurg Soc 2008;44(4):199.

78. Nanda A, Javalkar V, Zhang S, et al. Long term efficacy and patient satisfaction of microvascular decompression and gamma knife radiosurgery for trigeminal neuralgia. J Clin Neurosci 2015;22(5): 818–22.

79. Pollock BE, Schoeberl KA. Prospective comparison of posterior fossa exploration and stereotactic radiosurgery dorsal root entry zone target as primary surgery for patients with idiopathic trigeminal neuralgia. Neurosurgery 2010; 67(3):633–9.

80. Lopez BC, Hamlyn PJ, Zakrzewska JM. Systematic review of ablative neurosurgical techniques for the treatment of trigeminal neuralgia. Neurosurgery 2004;54(4):973–83.

Comparison of Prenatal and Postnatal Management of Patients with Myelomeningocele

CrossMark

Sergio Cavalheiro, MD, PhD[a],
Marcos Devanir Silva da Costa, MD, MSc[a,b],
Antonio Fernandes Moron, MD, PhD[c],
Jeffrey Leonard, MD[d],*

KEYWORDS

- Myelomeningocele • Fetal surgery • Spina bifida • Hydrocephalus • Chiari II malformation

KEY POINTS

- Myelomeningocele is a chronic disease that leads to significant disabilities, including sensory disturbances and weakness of the lower extremities.
- Prenatal ultrasonography and MRI have enabled earlier diagnosis of these patients.
- Prenatal myelomeningocele correction has shown good outcomes by reducing the ventriculoperitoneal shunt rate, and by improving ambulation status and mental development.
- Postnatal treatment of myelomeningocele continues to be the standard of care in many institutions.
- Antenatal myelomeningocele repair requires a multidisciplinary program not available in many institutions and should be discussed as a treatment option with new patients.

INTRODUCTION

Myelomeningocele (MMC) is a chronic disease that affects 0.3 to 0.72 per 1000 live-born and still-born babies in the United States.[1] MMC has a lifetime cost estimated at more than $620,000 in 2011 for each child born with MMC, which comprises direct medical costs, special education, caregiver needs, and loss of employment potential.[2]

MMC is an open neural tube defect that is fairly simple to correct, but consequences remain with patients for a lifetime. Patients with MMC often have morbidities related to lower limb sensory/motor impairment, ranging from weakness/hypoesthesia to paraplegia/anesthesia, bowel/bladder dysfunction, spinal and lower limb deformities (scoliosis, hip/ankle deformities, and club foot), and hydrocephalus.[3–5] Hydrocephalus affects as many as 85% of the patients with MMC operated after birth and also requires a lifetime of management.[3,6]

New imaging modalities (fetal ultrasonography and MRI) have facilitated prenatal diagnosis of MMC and have made possible prenatal MMC

Disclosure: The authors have nothing to disclose.
[a] Neurosurgery Department, Federal University of São Paulo–UNIFESP, Rua Pedro de Toledo, 715, 6th Floor, São Paulo, São Paulo 04024-001, Brazil; [b] Department of Pediatric Neurosurgery, Nationwide Children's Hospital, 700 Children's Drive, Columbus, OH 43205, USA; [c] Department of Obstetrics, Federal University of São Paulo–UNIFESP, Rua Pedro de Toledo, 715, 8th Floor, São Paulo, São Paulo 04024-001, Brazil; [d] Neurosurgery Department, Nationwide Children's Hospital, FB, Suite 4 A.2, 700 Children's Drive, Columbus, Ohio 43205, USA
* Corresponding author.
E-mail address: jeffrey.leonard@nationwidechildrens.org

Neurosurg Clin N Am 28 (2017) 439–448
http://dx.doi.org/10.1016/j.nec.2017.02.005
1042-3680/17/© 2017 Elsevier Inc. All rights reserved.

neurosurgery.theclinics.com

treatment, a key driver for the development of fetal surgery. Prenatal treatments were recently compared with the standard of care in a clinical trial.[3,4] However, this new treatment paradigm has generated several controversies, mainly regarding the maternal morbidity and premature birth of the fetus. This article reviews postnatal MMC repair, the features in the prenatal diagnosis, and prenatal MMC repair, and discusses the results and controversies concerning prenatal and postnatal MMC treatment.

POSTNATAL REPAIR OF MYELOMENINGOCELE

Despite the new emphasis on the antenatal correction of MMC recently published in the Management of Myelomeningocele Study (MOMS) trial,[3] postnatal repair of MMC continuous to be a standard of care in many institutions in the United States and around the world. It is important to highlight that, even as a standard of care, the postnatal repair of MMC has many difference among centers caring for the patients with MMC. A German study that enrolled 57 neurosurgery departments and 18 pediatric surgery departments surveyed the centers about management of open MMC in their hospitals. Significant differences in the therapeutic decisions were reported, including the type of delivery, timing to treat the MMC after birth, type of preoperative diagnostic image tool, type of prophylactic antibiotics, timing to treat hydrocephalus, and type of valve used to treat hydrocephalus.[7]

Guidelines regarding management of MMC currently do not exist. With the completion of the MOMS trial, prenatal repair should now be discussed with each newly diagnosed patient as a potential option for treatment. For those patients who will be repaired after birth, the first issue after the antenatal diagnosis of an MMC is the type of delivery. Many centers prefer the cesarean section as a route of delivery, advocating that this route is safer and protective to the neonate, the meningocele sac, and to the neural tissue/placode. However, there is no consensus to date because of the absence of a randomized clinical trial studying this question. One cohort study, conducted by Luthy and colleagues,[8] showed better motor functions at the age of 2 years for those patients delivered by cesarean section before labor compared with those delivered by vaginal route or cesarean section after labor. In contrast, other cohort studies designed to investigate the motor function after birth did not find any outcome difference between vaginal and cesarean section delivery.[9–13] Despite the

possible controversy, elective cesarean section remains attractive to many centers because it allows the scheduling of the MMC correction after birth and transforms a possible urgent surgery in an elective correction that benefits the newborn.

The timing of MMC repair has changed over the past 50 years. Before the 1960s, mortality and infection rates in patients with MMC were as high as 90% and in this scenario many neurosurgeons opted for conservative treatment with MMC defects left to heal by reepithelialization.[4,14] With introduction of the Holter valve to treat hydrocephalus, the mortality of patients with MMC decreased significantly. The neurologic impairment, which was until then considered a secondary issue, became more evident.

By the 1960s some researchers, concerned with the poor neurologic outcomes of patients with MMC, started to compare conservative versus operative repair of MMC. The first randomized clinical trial conducted by John and colleagues[14] enrolled 20 patients for each operative and nonoperative group, and the study had to be stopped because of improved outcomes for patients operated on within 48 hours. They had improved outcomes related to mortality, fewer wound infection, hydrocephalus, meningitis and ventriculitis, and muscle strength, and an improved hospital length of stay. Thus the investigators concluded that the MMC should be repaired as a surgical emergency.

Since then, many cohort and case series studies have reported an increase in the infection rates for those patients operated after 48 hours of life,[15] a decrease in the wound dehiscence and neurodevelopment delay at age 1 year for those patients operated immediately after birth,[16] and also an increase in infection rates and length of hospitalization for those patients operated after 24 hours of birth.[17] Thus the data suggest that the early repair of MMC is a goal to be achieved in order to improve patients' outcomes. Most of the cohort studies and the only randomized trial showed better results when the MMC was repaired within 48 hours of birth.[14–19] However, even the most aggressive treatment after birth has not shown a reduction in the hydrocephalus rate.[16]

Hydrocephalus in patients with MMC repaired after birth occurs at an approximate frequency of 82% at 12 months after birth.[3] The pathophysiology of hydrocephalus in the context of MMC and Chiari II malformation is complex and has not been well established. McLone and Knepper[20] proposed a theory that neurulation failure in the MMC leads to an open defect in the distal neural tube, creating a cerebrospinal fluid leakage that consequently causes a lack of distention of the rhombencephalic vesicles. This lack of distention in turn alters the inductive effect in the mesenchymal and endo-chondral bone formation of the posterior fossa, generating a small posterior fossa, a downward tonsils herniation, and a brainstem displacement, and thus the hydrocephalus in this context is related to the malformation of the cerebrospinal fluid pathways in the small posterior fossa.

Given the high rates of hydrocephalus related to MMC in patients undergoing postnatal correction, some studies were designed to assess the advantages associated with performing the MMC correction and implantation of the ventriculoperitoneal shunt in the same time. Although those studies have shown safety, low infection rates, and improved wound healing in patients with MMC,[21–24] limitations of this approach are that no study has identified a rate of hydrocephalus even close to 100%. Furthermore, patients undergoing ventriculoperitoneal shunt surgery are subject to a dysfunction rate that can be as high as 45.9% in the first year.[25] Despite being safe, the performance of 2 simultaneous operations is not a common practice because of a decreasing incidence of shunt placement in the MMC population. Therefore, there is not a preestablished best time to perform placement of a ventriculoperitoneal shunt. To standardize indications for ventriculoperitoneal shunt placement in the MOMS trial, specific criteria were defined and are listed here.[3]

At least 2 of the following are required for shunt placement:

- An increase in the greatest occipital-frontal circumference adjusted for the gestational age defined as crossing percentiles. Patients who cross centiles and subsequently plateau do not meet this criterion.
- A bulging fontanel (defined as above the bone assessed when the baby is in an upright position and not crying) or split sutures or sunsetting sign (eyes appear to look downward with the sclera prominent over the iris).
- Increasing ventricular measurements on consecutive imaging studies determined by increase in ratio of biventricular diameter to biparietal diameter according to the method of O'Hayon and colleagues.[26]
- Head circumference greater than the 95th percentile for gestational age.

At least 1 of the following criteria is required for shunt placement:

- Presence of marked syringomyelia (syrinx with expansion of spinal cord) with ventriculomegaly (undefined).
- Ventriculomegaly (undefined) and symptoms of Chiari malformation (stridor, swallowing difficulties, apnea, bradycardia).
- Persistent cerebrospinal fluid leakage from the MMC wound or bulging at the repair site.

Tulipan and colleagues[5] analyzed the prerandomization risks of patients in the MOMS trial and found that 25% of patients in the postnatal group presented with persistence of cerebrospinal fluid leakage or bulging of the wound as the criterion for placement of ventriculoperitoneal shunt compared with 1.1% of the intrauterine operated group, and this criterion accounted for 60% of the difference in the placing ventriculoperitoneal shunts between the two groups. In a different study, Chakraborty and colleagues[27] reported rates of ventriculoperitoneal shunt placement at 51.9% in patients operated for MMC after birth when they standardized criteria for shunt placement. They tolerated moderate and increasing ventricular dilatation, and treated the operative fistula wound as a local complication and not as a criterion for hydrocephalus. However, other investigators have reported that cerebrospinal fluid leakage in the MMC wound was a risk factor for meningitis or ventriculites.[28]

PRENATAL DIAGNOSIS OF MYELOMENINGOCELE

The routine use of two-dimensional prenatal ultrasonography has facilitated the prenatal diagnosis of MMC and rachischisis with increasing frequency. Accurate diagnosis of the disease and identification of the level of the lesion are now possible for counseling purposes. Ultrasonography is 90% sensitive and is often complimented by fetal MRI. Evaluation of the fetal spine by ultrasonography and cranial signs of spinal dysraphism can be evaluated from the 12th week of gestation. For the evaluation of the fetal spine, a full sweep in sagittal, coronal, and transverse sections of the spine is recommended, with a focus on vertebral bodies in the spinal canal and medulla.[29]

Two-dimensional prenatal ultrasonography in association with three-dimensional ultrasonography allows a detailed analysis of the spinal characteristics of MMC, such as the type of spinal dysraphism (meningocele, MMC, or rachischisis; **Fig. 1**), the anatomic level of the lesion (**Fig. 2**), alterations of the curvature of the spine, associated malformations of the spinal (syringomyelia and diastematomyelia), and the degree of herniation in the posterior fossa structures near the foramen magnum[30] (**Fig. 3**).

Cranial ultrasonography can be used to identify cranial features of MMC that include the

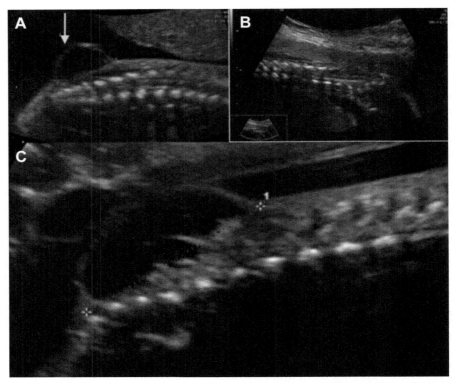

Fig. 1. Two-dimensional ultrasonography showing (*A*) meningocele (*arrow*), (*B*) rachischisis, (*C*) MMC with a neural tissue inside and the respective intraoperative view.

following: the lemon sign, which represents the so-called dry brain and features fetal intracranial hypotension (**Fig. 4**)[31,32]; ventriculomegaly assessed at the level of the atrium in the lateral ventricle (abnormal when >10 mm),[33] which is present in 70% to 90% of fetuses with an MMC (the characteristic pattern is colpocephaly); and the banana sign, which describes the echography findings in the axial plane of the cerebellar herniation through the foramen magnum (**Fig. 5**).[31,34] These 3 cranial signals have a specificity of 99% in MMC, but they may also be present in normal fetuses of obese mothers.[31]

Fig. 2. Two-dimensional ultrasonography. Counting of vertebral bodies by determining the 12th thoracic vertebra, which corresponds with the last rib.

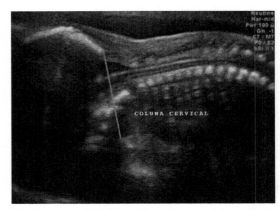

Fig. 3. The occipital-dens line, described to evaluate the degree of the brainstem and tonsil herniation into the cervical spine canal.

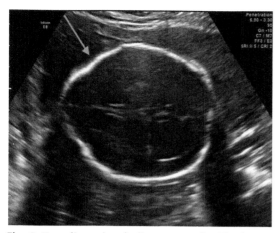

Fig. 4. Two-dimensional ultrasonography. The lemon sign: the skull in a shape of a lemon (*arrow*) because of the frontal scalloping of bone caused by intracranial hypotension.

Ultrasonography can also be used to infer the degree of impairment of the lower limbs in fetuses with MMC by identifying the presence of clubfoot and the degree of tropism of the lower limbs. It is possible to deduce the amount of fat that is replacing the skeletal muscle in the presence of severe paralysis of the lower limbs. When actively evaluated, the movement of the lower limbs can show a good prognosis compared with the presence of bilateral clubfeet. Notably, open dysraphism can produce involuntary movements of the fetus, leading to a false diagnosis.[35]

Prenatal Imaging Assessment: Fetal MRI

Fetal MRI is a complimentary diagnostic imaging modality to ultrasonography. MRI is performed

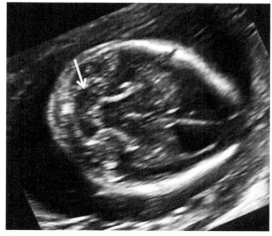

Fig. 5. The banana sign, which represents the inversion of the cerebellum curvature (*arrow*).

with ultrafast sequences to minimize the adverse effects of signs of maternal and fetal movements. T2-weighted (T2-W) images are enough for most of the information used for the diagnosis, including single-shot fast spin-echo or half-Fourier acquisition single-shot turbo spin-echo sequences at minimal slice thickness (2–4 mm). Gadolinium is not used as a contrast agent because is retained for a long period in the fetus–amniotic fluid system, and is not necessary for the diagnosis of MMC. The excellent soft tissue contrast resolution between the cord and the surrounding cerebrospinal fluid allows improved delineation of abnormal structures (**Fig. 6**).[36] This delineation is important for the detection of other closed spinal dysraphisms, such as lipomyelomeningocele, and other central nervous system malformations such as the callosal dysgenesis/hypogenesis, periventricular nodular heterotopy, cerebellar dysplasia, syringohydromyelia, and diastematomyelia.[37]

PRENATAL REPAIR OF MYELOMENINGOCELE

Fetal surgery requires the work of a multidisciplinary team (obstetrician, neurosurgeon, neonatologist, geneticist, anesthesiologist, nurse, physiotherapist, psychologist, and orthopedists, among others) in which each professional has a role and is interacting at all times of the treatment. Increased maternal risks are inherent to the procedure and the use of anesthetics, tocolytics, and other medications. Fetal surgeons should have the ability to correct anomalies in fetuses that are less than 27 weeks together with the capacity to maintain stable maternal and fetal hemodynamic conditions throughout the procedure. Prenatal repair of patients with MMC should occur between gestational age 19 and 27 weeks and 6 days, at a maternal age of at least 18 years, for Chiari type II spinal dysraphism ranging between T1 and S1, and for normal fetal karyotypes, with the cases that did not meet these criteria to be evaluated and discussed in a multidisciplinary forum before proceeding to surgery.

The initial experience of the Brazilian group shows that the results of the MOMs trial can be applied to create a highly successful program even outside the United States.[38] Obstetricians perform a 5-cm hysterotomy. After the hysterotomy, the fetus is positioned so that the neurosurgeon can perform correction of the MMC. The most important step is the release of the cord and the treatment of the tethered spinal cord. Often a fibrotic band is found while fixing the top part of the placode to the dura mater, which is called the cava ligament. This ligament is found in more than 90% of cases of MMC. Some

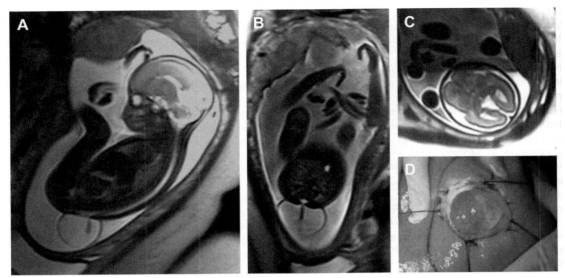

Fig. 6. T2-W MRI. (*A*) Large lumbosacral MMC with a spinal cord inside the herniary sac. (*B*) Coronal view showing the spinal dysraphism. (*C*) Colpocephalic aspect of the lateral ventricles. (*D*) Intraoperative view of the MMC.

investigators recommend using artificial grafts to close the dura mater.[39] This procedure is intended only to protect the neural tissue from the amniotic fluid and intrauterine trauma. After reconstruction of the placode to its original form, the dura and fascia are closed in a watertight fashion. In addition, the skin is closed with an absorbable continuous suture. After closure of the MMC, the fetus is released into the uterine cavity. The amniotic fluid is replaced and the uterus is closed.

Fetal neurosurgery entails the monitoring of the fetus from the moment of birth to the postnatal period. It is clear that the more delayed the delivery, the better the conditions of the newborn, but maternal health should be taken into consideration, particularly the quantity of the amniotic fluid and the thickness of the surgical scar. The rupture of amniotic membranes and the transition to oligohydramnios indicate the anticipation of labor, as well as the thinning of the uterine scar. If a thinning of the uterine scar is detected, early childbirth can prevent uterine rupture. Postoperative fetal monitoring includes observation of the MMC scar, calculation of ventricular size, and determination of the degree of both brainstem and tonsillar herniation.

Outcomes of Postnatal Versus Prenatal Myelomeningocele Correction

Recently the outcomes of postnatal and prenatal MMC correction were evaluated in the MOMS trial, which was terminated because of benefits in the prenatal group.[3] The objective of the MOMS trial

was to assess the results of intrauterine surgery compared with postnatal surgery. The primary end point of the MOMS trial was to analyze the fetal or neonatal mortality and the incidence of ventriculoperitoneal shunts until 1 year of age. The secondary end point was an evaluation of cognitive and motor development at 30 months of age. The main inclusion criteria were pregnancy, MMC from level T1 to S1, a gestational age between 19 and 25 weeks 6 days, a randomized and normal karyotype, and a maternal age of more than 18 years. The major exclusion criteria were fetal anomalies unrelated to MMC, severe kyphosis, risk of premature birth (including short cervix and previous preterm delivery), and placental abruption. The study showed a statistically significant reduction in incidence of hydrocephalus and need for ventriculoperitoneal shunts compared with the prenatal group (40% vs 82%). In addition, Tulipan and colleagues[5] in a recent update of the MOMS cohort reported that the main prenatal risk factor for the shunt placement was the ventricle size; fetuses with ventricle size less than 10 mm had 20% of shunt placement, those with ventricle size between 10 mm and up to 15 mm had 45.2%, and those with ventricles larger than 15 mm had 79% of shunt placement. Moreover, 42% of the prenatal group presented with an independent gait at 30 months of life compared with 21% in the postnatal group (P<.001). Chiari malformation II was reversed in 36% of the prenatal group compared with only 4% of the postnatal group; the symptomatic Chiari II index was 6% and 22%, respectively. Larger studies are required for a better understanding of the evolution of vesical and intestinal sphincteric function, in addition to sexual function in these patients. Fetal benefits should be evaluated from the perspective of increased maternal risk caused by the increased incidence of complications such as premature rupture of membranes (46%), premature birth (79%), and the observed mean gestational age at birth of 34.1 weeks in the fetal surgery group compared with 37.3 weeks in the postnatal surgery group. In addition, a uterine scar from a hysterotomy resulted in various complications, including varying degrees of weakness of the uterine wall in 25% of the women at birth, 9% partial rupture, and 1% total rupture of the uterine scar.

Although the MOMS trial used strict inclusion and exclusion criteria for its study patients, in everyday practice, clinicians tend to be less rigid. Patients with controlled hypertension, diabetes, and some types of autoimmune diseases, such as systemic lupus erythematosus, can undergo the procedures.

Surgery is not recommended in cases with kyphoscoliosis and injury above L1. Ventriculomegaly greater than 16 mm is a formal MOMS exclusion criterion. In the Brazilian case series (update of initial publication),[38] ventriculomegaly greater than 20 mm is a contraindication for prenatal repair of MMC. Many patients have colpocephaly but are not truly hydrocephalic. Five patients in our series had ventriculomegaly greater than 16 mm, and in 1 case there was a need for a ventricular shunt after birth. Age and weight are other important factors as well. For some patients with a body mass index greater than 35, the authors have also recommended surgery. In a series of 200 patients who underwent surgery for correction of MMC in utero in Santa Joana Hospital and Maternity Center of São Paulo, Brazil, and the Federal University of São Paulo (UNIFESP), Paulista Medical School (update of initial publication),[38] gestational age at operation ranged from 24 to 27 2/7 weeks (**Table 1**). Eighteen cases (9%) were born at less than 30 weeks of gestation, 74 (37%) cases were born between 30 and 34 weeks, 70 (35%) cases were born between 35 and 36 weeks, and 38 (19%) cases were born after 37 weeks. On average, the gestational age at birth was 34 weeks. Perinatal mortality occurred in 4 cases (2%), 2 of which were caused by chorioamnionitis, 1 was caused by a premature rupture of membranes, and another was caused by idiopathic bradycardia.

The mean birth weight was on average 2199 ± 571 g. Fourteen patients required a ventriculoperitoneal shunt up to 5 years later (7%), most cases required a shunt while still in the maternity unit (10 cases), and were all newborns born before 34 weeks. Significant changes were observed in the degree of hindbrain herniation; in our series, 160 (80%) cases did not present herniation, 28 (14%) cases showed a mild herniation, and 12 (6%) showed a moderate herniation. There were no cases of symptomatic Chiari. There was also an improvement of motor function compared with the anatomic level; 130 cases (65%) showed improvement by 1 or 2 levels, 40 cases (20%) remained unchanged, and 30 (15%) worsened. The motor function is very difficult to evaluate when comparing the anatomic with the motor levels. Rachischisis presented a better development than the MMC. Two patients needed to be submitted to reoperation because of a tethered cord, and in both cases the presence of epidermoid tumor was identified. One of the patients required 3 procedures and presented an extensive MMC from L2 to S2. Leal da Cruz and colleagues[40] analyzed a cohort of the first 51 patients and found that 93.7% had significantly less urinary tract dysfunction of high bladder pressure or incontinence. These results reveal the challenges that still have to be overcome in patients with MMC.

Moldenhauer and colleagues[41] in the Children's Hospital of Philadelphia in a post-MOMS study had 6 (6%) deaths in a cohort of 100 patients: 2 intrauterine fetal demises and 4 cases of neonatal demise. They reported a mean gestational age at birth of 34.3 weeks; 9 (9.4%) cases had a gestational age at birth of less than 30 weeks, 35 (36.4%) between 30 and 34 weeks, 26 (27.1%) between 35 and 36 weeks, and 26 (27.1%) at more than 36 weeks, which is comparable with the other 2 groups.

The newborns had a mean birth weight of 2415.5 g, 59 (71.1%) of them had no hindbrain herniation, 7 (8.4%) had mild herniation, and 13 (15.7%) had moderate/severe hindbrain herniation. Moreover, the investigators reported very good results regarding the difference between motor function and anatomic level: 44 (55%) patients had 1 or more levels better, 16 (32.5%) had no difference, and 10 (12.5%) had at least 1 level worse. Two patients (2.4%) were shunted before the discharge.

Zamlynski and colleagues[42] in a study comparing prenatal with postnatal treatments of spina bifida, had 2 (4.3%) mortalities in a cohort of 46 patients operated prenatally. Moreover, prenatally treated patients experienced a shunt rate of 27.8% compared with 80% in the postnatal group. **Table 1** compares the outcomes between the MOMS, the Children's hospital of philadelphia (CHOP), and the high-volume center in Brazil.

Table 1
Comparison of outcomes between prenatal and postnatal myelomeningocele repair

Period of Cohort Correction	MOMS Trial		HSJ-EPM/UNIFESP	CHOP
	Postnatal	Prenatal	Prenatal	Prenatal
Cases (N)	80	78	200	100
Perinatal death: N (%)	2 (2)[b]	2 (3)[b]	4 (2)	6 (6.1)[c]
Gestational age of birth (wk ± SD)	37.3 ± 1.1[a]	34.1 ± 3.1[a]	34	34.3
Gestational Age at Birth: N (%)				
<30 wk	0[a]	10 (13)[a]	18 (9)	9 (9.4)[c]
30–34 wk	4 (5)[a]	26 (33)[a]	74 (37)	35 (36.4)[c]
35–36 wk	8 (10)[a]	26 (33)[a]	70 (35)	26 (27.1)[c]
>36 wk	68 (85)[a]	16 (21)[a]	38 (19)	26 (27.1)[c]
Mean birth weight (g)	3039 ± 496[a]	2382 ± 688[a]	2199 ± 571	2415.5[c]
Placement of shunt: N (%)	66 (82)[a]	31 (40)[a]	14 (7)	2 (2.4)[d]
Degree of Hindbrain Herniation: N/Total N (%)				
None	3/69 (4)[a]	25/70 (36)[a]	160/200 (80)	59/83 (71.1)
Mild	20/69 (29)[a]	28/70 (40)[a]	28/200 (14)	7/83 (8.4)
Moderate	31/69 (45)[a]	13/70 (19)[a]	12/200 (6)	13/83 (15.7)
Severe	15/69 (22)[a]	4/70 (6)[a]	0	
Difference Between Motor Function and Anatomic Levels: N/total N (%)				
≥2 levels better	8/67 (12)[a]	20/62 (32)[a]	130/200 (65)	24/80 (30)
1 level better	6/67 (9)[a]	7/62 (11)[a]		20/80 (25)
No difference	17/67 (25)[a]	14/62 (23)[a]	20/200 (20)	26/80 (32.5)
1 level worse	17/67 (25)[a]	13/62 (21)[a]	30/200 (15)	9/80 (11.25)
≥2 levels worse	19/67 (28)[a]	8/62 (13)[a]		1/80 (1.25)

Abbreviations: CHOP, Children's hospital of philadelphia; HSJ-EPM/UNIFESP, Santa Joana Hospital and Maternity Center of São Paulo, Brazil and the UNIFESP, Paulista Medical School; SD, standard deviation.
 [a] This highlights the statistical difference between groups in the MOMS trial (at least $P<.05$).
 [b] No statistical difference between the groups in the MOMS trial.
 [c] Prevalence based on 96 cases in the CHOP.
 [d] Shunt rate before hospital discharge.

A French pilot study, designed to establish the prenatal repair in a reference center, found 22 patients eligible for prenatal surgery. However, most of the couples opted for the termination of the gestation; in this way, from those 22 patients, only 3 were successfully operated intrauterus and another 4 patients were operated postnatally.[43] This finding shows that prenatal surgery for MMC can be established in different countries, but the culture, the law, the religion, and the ability to interrupt the gestation may affect management of the disease and increase the volume of patients in reference centers.

Future Perspectives of Myelomeningocele Treatment

Minimally invasive surgeries that are performed using endoscopic techniques are very promising. However, to date the literature has not supported this procedure. None of the observed outcomes have been superior to fetal open surgical techniques. The fetoscopic correction of MMC is limited in providing a watertight closure, because it is based on a fixation of an artificial membrane that protects the placode, preventing development of a cerebrospinal fluid fistula. Another disadvantage of this technique is the impossibility of untethering of the spinal cord, which is a crucial step an MMC correction. Joeyeux and colleagues[44] in a recent systematic review showed that the perinatal mortality in the fetoscopic correction groups varied from 7.8% to 20%, with other outcomes comparable except for uterine thinning or dehiscence, which was less frequent in the fetoscopic group; the time of procedure, which was higher in the fetoscopic groups; and the Chiari malformation decompression, which was not reported in the fetoscopic groups; as well as the ability to walk at 1 year.

SUMMARY

MMC is a complex disease, and treatment has been a challenge for many years. The most recent studies on MMC point to earlier approaches during fetal life as a valuable alternative to reduce the hydrocephalus rates and improve motor patterns of these patients. A multidisciplinary approach in a quaternary center is required and can be created in large centers outside the United States, as shown by the results from the Brazilian center. A large volume of patients is required as well as detailed reporting of patient outcomes because of the increased risk to mothers and the increase in morbidity related to premature birth.

REFERENCES

1. Cragan JD, Roberts HE, Edmonds LD, et al. Surveillance for anencephaly and spina bifida and the impact of prenatal diagnosis–United States, 1985-1994. MMWR CDC Surveill Summ 1995;44(4):1–13.

2. Yi Y, Lindemann M, Colligs A, et al. Economic burden of neural tube defects and impact of prevention with folic acid: a literature review. Eur J Pediatr 2011;170(11):1391–400.

3. Adzick NS, Thom EA, Spong CY, et al. A randomized trial of prenatal versus postnatal repair of myelomeningocele. N Engl J Med 2011;364(11):993–1004.

4. Keller BA, Farmer DL. Fetal surgery for myelomeningocele: history, research, clinical trials, and future directions. Minerva Pediatr 2015;67(4):341–56.

5. Tulipan N, Wellons JC 3rd, Thom EA, et al. Prenatal surgery for myelomeningocele and the need for cerebrospinal fluid shunt placement. J Neurosurg Pediatr 2015;16(6):613–20.

6. Tamburrini G, Frassanito P, Iakovaki K, et al. Myelomeningocele: the management of the associated hydrocephalus. Childs Nerv Syst 2013;29(9):1569–79.

7. Mauer UM, Jahn A, Unterreithmeir L, et al. Survey on current postnatal surgical management of myelomeningocele in Germany. J Neurol Surg A Cent Eur Neurosurg 2016;77(6):489–94.

8. Luthy DA, Wardinsky T, Shurtleff DB, et al. Cesarean section before the onset of labor and subsequent motor function in infants with meningomyelocele diagnosed antenatally. N Engl J Med 1991;324(10):662–6.

9. Cochrane D, Aronyk K, Sawatzky B, et al. The effects of labor and delivery on spinal cord function and ambulation in patients with meningomyelocele. Childs Nerv Syst 1991;7(6):312–5.

10. Cuppen I, Eggink AJ, Lotgering FK, et al. Influence of birth mode on early neurological outcome in infants with myelomeningocele. Eur J Obstet Gynecol Reprod Biol 2011;156(1):18–22.

11. Greene S, Lee PS, Deibert CP, et al. The impact of mode of delivery on infant neurologic outcomes in myelomeningocele. Am J Obstet Gynecol 2016;215(4):495.e1-11.

12. Lewis D, Tolosa JE, Kaufmann M, et al. Elective cesarean delivery and long-term motor function or ambulation status in infants with meningomyelocele. Obstet Gynecol 2004;103(3):469–73.

13. Merrill DC, Goodwin P, Burson JM, et al. The optimal route of delivery for fetal meningomyelocele. Am J Obstet Gynecol 1998;179(1):235–40.

14. John W, Sharrard W, Zachary RB, et al. A controlled trial of immediate and delayed closure of spina bifida cystica. Arch Dis Child 1963;38(197):18–22.

15. Rodrigues AB, Krebs VL, Matushita H, et al. Short-term prognostic factors in myelomeningocele patients. Childs Nerv Syst 2016;32(4):675–80.

16. Pinto FC, Matushita H, Furlan AL, et al. Surgical treatment of myelomeningocele carried out at 'time zero' immediately after birth. Pediatr Neurosurg 2009;45(2):114–8.

17. Attenello FJ, Tuchman A, Christian EA, et al. Infection rate correlated with time to repair of open neural tube defects (myelomeningoceles): an institutional and national study. Childs Nerv Syst 2016;32(9):1675–81.

18. Lorber J. Results of treatment of myelomeningocele. An analysis of 524 unselected cases, with special reference to possible selection for treatment. Dev Med Child Neurol 1971;13(3):279–303.

19. Steinbok P, Irvine B, Cochrane DD, et al. Long-term outcome and complications of children born with meningomyelocele. Childs Nerv Syst 1992;8(2):92–6.

20. McLone DG, Knepper PA. The cause of Chiari II malformation: a unified theory. Pediatr Neurosci 1989;15(1):1–12.

21. Bell WO, Arbit E, Fraser RA. One-stage meningomyelocele closure and ventriculoperitoneal shunt placement. Surg Neurol 1987;27(3):233–6.

22. Chadduck WM, Reding DL. Experience with simultaneous ventriculo-peritoneal shunt placement and myelomeningocele repair. J Pediatr Surg 1988;23(10):913–6.

23. Epstein NE, Rosenthal AD, Zito J, et al. Shunt placement and myelomeningocele repair: simultaneous vs sequential shunting. Review of 12 cases. Childs Nerv Syst 1985;1(3):145–7.

24. Hubballah MY, Hoffman HJ. Early repair of myelomeningocele and simultaneous insertion of ventriculoperitoneal shunt: technique and results. Neurosurgery 1987;20(1):21–3.

25. Caldarelli M, Di Rocco C, La Marca F. Shunt complications in the first postoperative year in children with meningomyelocele. Childs Nerv Syst 1996;12(12):748–54.

26. O'Hayon BB, Drake JM, Ossip MG, et al. Frontal and occipital horn ratio: A linear estimate of ventricular

size for multiple imaging modalities in pediatric hydrocephalus. Pediatr Neurosurg 1998;29(5):245–9.

27. Chakraborty A, Crimmins D, Hayward R, et al. Toward reducing shunt placement rates in patients with myelomeningocele. J Neurosurg Pediatr 2008; 1(5):361–5.

28. Clemmensen D, Rasmussen MM, Mosdal C. A retrospective study of infections after primary VP shunt placement in the newborn with myelomeningocele without prophylactic antibiotics. Childs Nerv Syst 2010;26(11):1517–21.

29. Coleman BG, Langer JE, Horii SC. The diagnostic features of spina bifida: the role of ultrasound. Fetal Diagn Ther 2015;37(3):179–96.

30. de Sa Barreto EQ, Moron AF, Milani HJ, et al. The occipitum-dens line: the purpose of a new ultrasonographic landmark in the evaluation of the relationship between the foetal posterior fossa structures and foramen magnum. Childs Nerv Syst 2015; 31(5):729–33.

31. Nicolaides KH, Campbell S, Gabbe SG, et al. Ultrasound screening for spina bifida: cranial and cerebellar signs. Lancet 1986;2(8498):72–4.

32. Nyberg DA, Mack LA, Hirsch J, et al. Abnormalities of fetal cranial contour in sonographic detection of spina bifida: evaluation of the "lemon" sign. Radiology 1988;167(2):387–92.

33. Cardoza JD, Goldstein RB, Filly RA. Exclusion of fetal ventriculomegaly with a single measurement: the width of the lateral ventricular atrium. Radiology 1988;169(3):711–4.

34. Campbell J, Gilbert WM, Nicolaides KH, et al. Ultrasound screening for spina bifida: cranial and cerebellar signs in a high-risk population. Obstet Gynecol 1987;70(2):247–50.

35. Sival DA, van Weerden TW, Vles JS, et al. Neonatal loss of motor function in human spina bifida aperta. Pediatrics 2004;114(2):427–34.

36. Griffiths PD, Widjaja E, Paley MN, et al. Imaging the fetal spine using in utero MR: diagnostic accuracy and impact on management. Pediatr Radiol 2006; 36(9):927–33.

37. Simon EM. MRI of the fetal spine. Pediatr Radiol 2004;34(9):712–9.

38. Hisaba WJ, Cavalheiro S, Almodim CG, et al. Intrauterine myelomeningocele repair postnatal results and follow-up at 3.5 years of age–initial experience from a single reference service in Brazil. Childs Nerv Syst 2012;28(3):461–7.

39. Watanabe M, Jo J, Radu A, et al. A tissue engineering approach for prenatal closure of myelomeningocele with gelatin sponges incorporating basic fibroblast growth factor. Tissue Eng Part A 2010; 16(5):1645–55.

40. Leal da Cruz M, Liguori R, Garrone G, et al. Categorization of bladder dynamics and treatment after fetal myelomeningocele repair: first 50 cases prospectively assessed. J Urol 2015;193(5 Suppl): 1808–11.

41. Moldenhauer JS, Soni S, Rintoul NE, et al. Fetal myelomeningocele repair: the post-MOMS experience at the Children's Hospital of Philadelphia. Fetal Diagn Ther 2015;37(3):235–40.

42. Zamlynski J, Olejek A, Koszutski T, et al. Comparison of prenatal and postnatal treatments of spina bifida in Poland–a non-randomized, single-center study. J Matern Fetal Neonatal Med 2014;27(14):1409–17.

43. Friszer S, Dhombres F, Di Rocco F, et al. Preliminary results from the French study on prenatal repair for fetal myelomeningoceles (the PRIUM study). J Gynecol Obstet Biol Reprod (Paris) 2016;45(7): 738–44 [in French].

44. Joyeux L, Engels AC, Russo FM, et al. Fetoscopic versus open repair for spina bifida aperta: a systematic review of outcomes. Fetal Diagn Ther 2016; 39(3):161–71.

Index

Note: Page numbers of article titles are in **boldface** type.

A

5-Aminolevulinic acid, for glioma visualization, 403
Aneurysm(s)
    small incidental, treatment of, **389–396**
    subarachnoid, flow diversion after, **375–388**
Aneurysm Study of Pipeline in an Observational
    Registry (ASPIRe), 386
Anterior cervical discectomy, 332–333
Anterior lumbar interbody fusions, 332–333
Antiplatelet therapy, flow diversion and, 377, 385
Arthrodesis, bone morphogenic protein for, **331–334**
ASPIRe (Aneurysm Study of Pipeline in an
    Observational Registry), 386
Aspirin, flow diversion and, 377
Astrocytomas, fibrillary, 402–403

B

Back pain
    in spinal deformity with radiculopathy, **341–347**
    sacroiliac fusion for, **301–320**
Balloon compression, for trigeminal neuralgia, 432
Blister aneurysms, 385
Bone morphogenic protein, for spinal surgery,
    331–334
Bupivacaine, for sacroiliac joint dysfunction, 302, 316
Burr holes, for moyamoya disease, 365–372

C

Cage placement, for sacroiliac fusion, 306–307
Chiari malformation decompression, 446
Clipping, microsurgical, for incidental aneurysms,
    389–396
Clopidogrel, flow diversion and, 377
Cloward bone plugs, for sacroiliac joint
    dysfunction, 317
Coflex interspinous spacers, 323
Coil treatment, for aneurysms, 391–395
Coiling-assisted flow diversion, 386
Compression, balloon, for trigeminal neuralgia, 432
Compression test, for sacroiliac joint dysfunction,
    303, 315–316
Computed tomography
    for sacroiliac dysfunction, 308
    for stroke, 351
Confocal microscopy, for gliomas, 403
Cryotherapy, for sacroiliac joint dysfunction, 316

D

Decompression
    for lumbar spinal stenosis, 324
    for scoliosis, **335–339**
    for spinal deformity with radiculopathy, **341–347**
    for trigeminal neuralgia, 429–431
Decompressive craniectomy, for stroke, **349–360**
DESTINY trials, 350–353
Direct bypass technique, for moyamoya disease,
    362–365, 370–372
Distraction maneuver, for sacroiliac joint dysfunction,
    303, 315–316

E

Encepaloduroarteriosynangiosis, 365–372
Encephalomyosynangiosis, 365–372
Endovascular treatment
    for aneurysmal subarachnoid hemorrhage,
    375–388
    for incidental aneurysms, **389–396**

F

FABER maneuvers, 301, 314–315
Femoral shear (thigh thrust) test, for sacroiliac joint
    dysfunction, 303, 315–316
Fetal surgery, for myelomeningocele, 443–446
Finnish Lumbar Spinal Research Group, **321–330**
Flow diversion, after subarachnoid hemorrhage,
    375–388
    case studies of, 379–380
    coiling-assisted, 386
    definition of, 377
    patient selection for, 377
    results of, 378–386
    shield technology with, 386
    technique for, 377–378
Fluorescence imaging, for gliomas, 403
Foraminotomy, for scoliosis, 338
Fortin finger test, for sacroiliac joint dysfunction,
    315–316
Functional mapping, for gliomas, 401–402

G

Gaenslen maneuver, for sacroiliac joint dysfunction,
    304, 315–316

neurosurgery.theclinics.com

Galveston technique, for sacroiliac fusion, 310
Genetic factors, in gliomas, 398
Gillet maneuver, for sacroiliac joint dysfunction, 315–316
Glioblastoma(s), 402–403
Glioblastoma multiforme, recurrent, reoperation for, literature review of, **407–428**
Gliomas, incidental, **397–406**
Glycerol rhizotomy, for trigeminal neuralgia, 432

H

HAMLET trial, 350–354
HeADDFIRST trial, 350–354
Hemicraniectomy, for stroke, **349–360**
    hemorrhagic, 356–357
    ischemic, 350–356
Hemorrhage, subarachnoid, flow diversion after, **375–388**
Hemorrhagic stroke, hemicraniectomy for, 356–357
Hydrocephalus, treatment of, 440–446

I

IDH1 protein defects, in gliomas, 398
Incidental aneurysms, treatment of, **389–396**
Indirect bypass technique, for moyamoya disease, 365–372
Infratentorial stroke, hemicraniectomy for, 354–356
Instrumentation-induced fusion, for spinal surgery, **331–334**
International Retrospective Study of Pipeline Embolism Device, 386
International Subarachnoid Aneurysm Trial, **375–388**
Interspinous spacers, for lumbar spinal stenosis, **321–330**
Intraarticular injection, for sacroiliac joint dysfunction, 302, 316
Intracerebral hemorrhage, 356–357
Ischemic stroke, hemicraniectomy for, 350–356

K

Kyphosis, radiculopathy with, **341–347**

L

Laminectomy, for scoliosis, 336–338
Lemon sign, in myelomeningocele, 442
Low back pain, sacroiliac fusion for, **301–320**
Low-grade gliomas, **397–406**
Lumbar radiculopathy, with degenerative scoliosis, **335–339**
Lumbar spinal stenosis, interspinous spacers for, **321–330**

M

Magnetic resonance imaging
    for gliomas, 398–399
    for moyamoya disease, 362
    for myelomeningocele, 441, 443
Maine Lumbar Spine Research Group, 322
Malignant stroke, 350, 354
Malignant transformation, of gliomas, 402–403
Management of Myelomeningocele Study (MOMS), 440–446
Mannitol, for stroke, 351
Material-induced fusion, for spinal surgery, **331–334**
Microsurgical clipping, for incidental aneurysms, **389–396**
Microsurgical resection, for gliomas, 399–401
Microvascular decompression, for trigeminal neuralgia, 429–431
MOMS (Management of Myelomeningocele Study), 440–446
Moyamoya disease, **362–374**
    epidemiology of, 361
    evaluation of, 362
    nonsurgical treatment of, 362
    pathophysiology of, 362
    surgical treatment of, 362–372
Myelomeningocele, **439–448**
    epidemiology of, 439
    postnatal repair of, 440–441, 444–446
    prenatal diagnosis of, 441–443
    prenatal repair of, 443–446

N

National Institutes of Health
    Recurrent GBM Scale, 417
    stroke scale, 351
Nerve ablation, for sacroiliac joint dysfunction, 316
Neural tube defects. See Myelomeningocele.
Neuralgia, trigeminal, **429–438**
Neurogenic claudication, interspinous spacers for, **321–330**

O

Oligodendrogliomas, 402–403
Omental transposition, for moyamoya disease, 367–372
Osmotherapy, for stroke, 351

P

p53 protein defects, in gliomas, 398
Pain
    back, sacroiliac fusion for, **301–320**
    in trigeminal neuralgia, **429–438**
    radicular, 314

Painter technique, for sacroiliac joint dysfunction, 317
Percutaneous treatments, microvascular, 431–433
PHASES score, 391
Pial synangiosis, 365–372
Pipeline for Uncoilable or Failed Aneurysm trial, 386
Positron emission tomography, for gliomas, 398–399
Posterior fossa stroke, hemicraniectomy for, 354–356
Proton magnetic resonance spectroscopy, for
    gliomas, 398

R

Radicular pain, versus sacroiliac joint pain, 314
Radiculopathy
    lumbar, with degenerative scoliosis, **335–339**
    spinal deformity with, **341–347**
Radiofrequency ablation, for sacroiliac joint
    dysfunction, 316–317
Radiofrequency rhizotomy, for trigeminal
    neuralgia, 431
Radiosurgery, stereotactic, for trigeminal neuralgia,
    432–433
Resection
    for glioblastoma multiforme, literature review of,
        407–428
    for gliomas, 399–401
Revascularization, for moyamoya disease, 362–372
Rhizotomy, for trigeminal neuralgia, 431–433
Ribbon encepaloduroarteriomyosynangiosis,
    365–372

S

Sacroiliac fusion
    for low back pain, **301–320**
    revision of, 305–308
Scoliosis, radiculopathy with, **335–339, 341–347**
Screw fixation, for sacroiliac fusion, 305
Shunt, for hydrocephalus, 440–446
Small aneurysms, treatment of, **389–396**
Smith-Petersen approach, 304, 317
Spina bifida. *See* Myelomeningocele.
Spinal fusion
    for low back pain, **301–320**
    for spinal deformity with radiculopathy, **341–347**
Spinal stenosis, radiculopathy with, **341–347**

Split duro-encephalosynangiosis, 365–372
SPORT (Spine Patient Outcomes Research Trial), 322
Steal phenomenon, in moyamoya disease, 362
Stereotactic biopsy, for gliomas, 399
Stereotactic radiosurgery, for trigeminal neuralgia,
    432–433
Stroke
    hemicraniectomy for, **349–360**
        hemorrhagic, 356–357
        ischemic, 350–356
    in moyamoya disease, 362
Strokectomy, 355
Subarachnoid hemorrhage, flow diversion after,
    375–388
Superficial temporal artery to middle cerebral artery
    bypass technique, for moyamoya disease,
    362–365, 370–372
Supratentorial stroke, 350–354, 357

T

TERT promoter defects, in gliomas, 398
Thigh thrust, for sacroiliac joint dysfunction, 303,
    315–316
Titanium rods, for sacroiliac fusion, 304–305
Trigeminal neuralgia, **429–438**

U

Ultrasonography, for myelomeningocele, 441–443
Unruptured aneurysms, treatment of, **389–396**

V

Ventriculoperitoneal shunt, for hydrocephalus,
    440–446
Ventriculostomy, for stroke, 354–356

W

Wallis interspinous spacers, 322

X

X-Stop Interspinous Process Decompression
    System, 322–326

Moving?

Make sure your subscription moves with you!

To notify us of your new address, find your **Clinics Account Number** (located on your mailing label above your name), and contact customer service at:

Email: journalscustomerservice-usa@elsevier.com

800-654-2452 (subscribers in the U.S. & Canada)
314-447-8871 (subscribers outside of the U.S. & Canada)

Fax number: 314-447-8029

Elsevier Health Sciences Division
Subscription Customer Service
3251 Riverport Lane
Maryland Heights, MO 63043

ELSEVIER

Printed and bound by CPI Group (UK) Ltd, Croydon, CR0 4YY

13/05/2025

01869712-0002